Permission
to Come
Home

Permission to Come Home

Reclaiming
Mental Health as
Asian Americans

JENNY T. WANG, PhD

balance

NEW YORK BOSTON

Balance
Hachette Book Group
1290 Avenue of the Americas, New York, NY 10104
gcp-balance.com
twitter.com/gcpbalance

First Edition: May 2022

Balance is an imprint of Grand Central Publishing. The Balance name and
logo are trademarks of Hachette Book Group, Inc.

The publisher is not responsible for websites (or their content) that are not
owned by the publisher.

The Hachette Speakers Bureau provides a wide range of authors for speaking
events. To find out more, go to www.hachettespeakersbureau.com or
call (866) 376-6591.

Library of Congress Cataloging-in-Publication Data
Names: Wang, Jenny T., author.
Title: Permission to come home : reclaiming mental health as Asian
Americans / Jenny T. Wang, PhD.
Description: First Edition. | New York, NY : Balance, 2022. | Includes
bibliographical references. |
Identifiers: LCCN 2021053689 | ISBN 9781538708002 (hardcover) |
ISBN 9781538708026 (ebook)
Subjects: LCSH: Asian Americans—Mental health—United States. |
Immigrants—Mental health—United States. | Minorities—Mental
Health—United States. | Self-care, Health.
Classification: LCC RC451.5.A75 W36 2022 |
DDC 362.2089/95073—dc23/eng/20220107
LC record available at https://lccn.loc.gov/2021053689

ISBNs: 978-1-5387-0800-2 (hardcover); 978-1-5387-0802-6 (ebook)

Printed in the United States of America

LSC-C

Printing 1, 2022

To Evie and Theo: I am a better human because of you both. May you one day pick up this book and embark on this journey too.

To 阿公 (Grandpa): I miss you. Thank you for watching over me as I wrote this book. I will see you again soon.

Contents

Introduction

People often ask me if I had personal mental health experiences that led to my interest in the field of psychology. Sometimes it feels as though my path would make more sense if a mental health crisis or major trauma had devastated my life, spurring a deep curiosity in suffering and healing. I have no such major event to recount, but rather a long pilgrimage of unlearning and transformation to become a better mother, wife, psychologist, and human being. I have come to realize that mental health permeates the many intimate spaces of our lives. Our suffering and well-being do not exist solely in overcoming major crises or managing diagnoses, but also within the conversations held behind closed doors, in the tears we shed alone in the shower, and in the deep emotions that we cannot ignore despite our best efforts.

The stigma against mental health is not only carried by Asian communities; it is pervasive in most cultures. Often, mental health concerns are attributed to temporary stressors, personality quirks, lack of willpower or strength, or poor life choices. When we admit that we are struggling, as all humans do, we are frequently shamed and told to "get over it" or "just stop thinking about it." The harm that this societal stigma causes to those courageously seeking help is incalculable.

This book is neither a research text nor a prescriptive how-to. It is also not a book describing mental health disorders or how to address them. It is an invitation for you, the reader, to take a journey with me, through the different spaces in your life that might be calling for your attention. To unpack the stories and narratives that might impact us, as members of Asian diasporas and children of immigrants, and that shape our mental health in profound ways. To wade through our painful experiences in order to understand how that pain has shaped us. And finally, to draw you closer to home, a space that perhaps has eluded many of us for a long time. A place of acceptance, belonging, healing, and freedom. What if our community invested in the individual transformation that could give way to communal and collective healing? I eagerly wait for this day, though I know I probably will be long gone when that day comes—which is why I hope you will join me in this journey of metamorphosis. Because this work of inner healing, relational reconciliation, and identity integration has the power to transform generations after us. I cannot even begin to imagine what is possible if we all committed to healing and prioritizing our mental health as a community.

While this book is written from the lens of experiences impacting Asian diasporas, it is important to mention that Asian Americans and broader Asian diasporic communities are vast and reflect many distinct ethnicities and people groups. It is impossible to fully capture the lived experiences of all Asian diasporas within a single book or even collection of texts. Here I speak from my own experiences, as an East Asian woman with my own privileges and marginalities, and from the shared experiences of my many Asian American clients, who have been shaped into anonymous and fictionalized composites to protect their confidentiality and privacy. Despite the wide range of experiences and stories across Asian diasporas, I do believe some commonalities run across ethnic and cultural lines through our shared experience of immigration to Western culture and some similarities in cultural values. It is these common threads that I share throughout this book, fully acknowledging that not all Asian diasporas will resonate with every example.

In order to write this book, I had to personally embark on the same voyage that I am inviting you into. Each chapter challenged me to question all my assumptions about my life, to upend all the falsehoods that trapped me, and to act in accordance with the values and life that I dreamed of living. This process was painful, stirred up so many of my fears, and forced me to face much of my personal and intergenerational pain, but it also freed me of the spaces that haunted me for most of my life. Please know that this work, identity work, may activate parts of your life that you may have worked hard to protect against and avoid for many years. So be gentle and kind with yourself in the process. I encourage you to draw upon the strength and resilience of your ancestors, supportive friends, family, or a mental health professional, if one is accessible to you, as you begin this difficult, but important work. Keep a notebook or journal nearby to take notes and complete some of the exercises you'll find in the book.

In the end, I hope this book is just the beginning for you. A start to new ways of thinking about your life, relating to others, and understanding, in a deep way, how immeasurably valuable you are and how much this world needs you to exist in full, authentic form. My hope is that you will return to chapters of this book in different seasons of your life to help you question, ponder, and explore your innermost needs and remind yourself that you deserve to live a life beyond your wildest dreams. All you need to do is to choose to step off the well-marked path.

Are you ready to join me? Let's get started.

CHAPTER 1

Permission to Question

When a great ship is in harbor and moored, it is safe, there can be no doubt. But that is not what great ships are built for.

—Clarissa Pinkola Estés

Be safe. Stay safe. For most of my life, these were the words with which I walked my path. Safety was the priority in almost every decision and encounter. As Asian immigrants, my parents came to the United States alone. With a tenuous grasp of English, they were terrified to even answer the phone in their early days, and safety was the first and most basic need in their life. My sister and I were constantly reminded to be safe, play it safe, and stay safe. For my parents, safety was the most important part of building stability in a foreign country. It makes perfect sense why they would instill the same value of safety in us.

In an effort to help me, people in my life thought giving me a map to follow would make things easier. The map had specific stopping points: Study hard. Get a degree. Get a job. Get married. Have children. Raise children. Retire. Die. No detours. No shortcuts. No unmarked trails. People said, "Stay on this path and it will keep you safe. But if you dare to veer off the clearly marked trail, we may not be there to save you from the lurking danger.

You'll be on your own." So, I took the map and started on this journey, believing every clearly marked path was all there was. Every mile marker served as confirmation that I was on the right route. I rarely questioned whether it was what I wanted or what I believed was right for me. Honestly, it was easier to play it safe and follow the map. Doing so involved less conflict with others. The rules were clearly written. It was easy to see where the goalposts were and how long it would take to get there. There were constant rewards for being obedient and compliant. All the pats on the back kept me fueled for the next leg of the journey.

Staying on this path also meant that I stayed comfortable, never stretching too far to the point of discomfort or taking major risks that might result in failure. It was a reasonable way to live, right? This was what my Taiwanese parents worked hard to provide for me, wasn't it? Along the way, I started adding my own notes to the map. When exciting but scary opportunities popped up, I added in my own limits, rules, and restrictions to protect me from taking these potentially dangerous detours. And each time I would think to myself, *Whew. Catastrophe averted! Good job staying safe, Jenny.* Another pat on the back.

But once in a while there would be moments—when everything was quiet, when I wasn't distracting myself with getting to the next mile marker—when I would notice, deep in my gut, a stirring. A wondering. A question. Is this all there is? Is this what I want? After following all the rules and staying inside the lines, is this the reward? Is this it?

Maybe this is where you are right now. You have slowed down or hit a wall. You have tried to silence that stirring because it would just be easier to stay on the map. But you also can no longer imagine staying the same. You are at a point of questioning.

You are wondering if you should veer onto that unmarked path. And it is terrifying you. Here, I invite you to begin our journey together.

This book has no easy answers. Instead, it is filled with questions—questions I have asked myself over the years and questions I, as a psychologist, have witnessed my clients struggle with in search of a more authentic and empowered life, as members of Asian diasporas and children of immigrants. I must warn you that this identity work is hard. It is not comfortable, it may cause friction in your relationships, it may have you questioning whether you really know what you want, and it may leave you with a lot of uncertainty. This is the price of stepping off the well-marked path. But this is also the price of perhaps finally allowing yourself to discover who you are apart from the expectations of others.

Each chapter encourages you to give yourself permission to show up differently and release yourself from unwritten expectations, mindsets, or rules you may have picked up from your roadmap of life, and from ways of thinking that might be keeping you from living with freedom, empowerment, and connection. The goal is to name these unwritten mindsets and bring them to your awareness so that you can see their impact on your daily life. Awareness is key. With awareness, we can change patterns and quite possibly the entire trajectory of our lives.

———— **REST STOP** ————

Take a moment and create some space. When you are quiet and still, do you notice an area of wondering or stirring in your life, or an area of your life that feels misaligned or disconnected? What thoughts and emotions live in that space? Be gentle and curious with that part of yourself.

QUESTION EVERYTHING

In this first chapter, I invite you to question everything. Give yourself permission to question that stirring and rumbling within you. Give yourself permission to wonder why things may feel off, disconnected, or unsatisfying. You are allowed to feel these things, and, in fact, these feelings are giving you clues about your life. These questions are encouraging you to explore parts of yourself that might need your attention, parts that you may have silenced or forgotten along the way and that do not want to conform neatly to the map that you were handed early on in your life.

As a child of Asian immigrants, actively questioning parts of my life has been quite difficult. Sometimes the very act of questioning authority, rules, or the status quo can be seen as disrespectful or dishonoring to our parents and their sacrifices. Questioning can trigger emotions of guilt or shame. We might feel like questioning is a sign that we are ungrateful for what has been offered to us, especially when staying silent and not raising questions has been praised or encouraged. It makes sense why questioning parts of our lives can bring up so much conflict internally and externally.

But as we start this identity work, we must ask ourselves, "What is the cost of not questioning? What is the cost of remaining unaware of what impacts our thoughts, emotions, and choices?" When we do not question the powerful frameworks that influence our lives, we lack awareness. Without awareness, we lose agency and freedom of choice over our lives. When we lack awareness, we react out of impulse or instinct to triggers and situations, instead of responding with intention. We replay old dynamics and maintain patterns of living that keep us stuck.

An important note here: I am not asking you to question these frameworks so that you can discard all elements of your upbringing and culture. In fact, just the opposite. In the process of asking, I am hoping you can embrace the family and cultural elements that make you feel strong, connected, and empowered, and make you uniquely you, while also releasing yourself from elements that might make you feel lesser than, restricted, or powerless. I am encouraging you to evaluate the frameworks that are important to you and consciously decide if and how you want to apply them to your life. Questioning actually means being curious long enough to wonder whether this way of thinking or living is ultimately working for us.

The rest of this chapter will explore areas of questioning that might impact you, as a child of an Asian diasporas. But these are not the only spaces of questioning that exist. In fact, I hope your questioning will extend far beyond these spaces. Your specific areas of questioning may be subtle but powerful forces. They may sometimes be historical, cultural, or structural in nature. They might feel like large roadblocks that divide spaces and try to dictate where you can and cannot enter. They can feel massive enough that you seem to run into them again and again, no matter how much insight you gain or how hard you try to push through them. They might also trigger deep insecurity, fear, guilt, or doubt.

However, they may also be spaces in which you might begin to gain more freedom once you acknowledge their presence in your life. Time and again, I have witnessed clients begin to see these structures and acknowledge how they hinder them from building an authentic life. I have seen people decide that rigidly adhering to some of these ideas kept them stuck, unable to feel empowered over parts of their lives. As you work through this book, you will begin to question some of these themes for yourself and, I hope, remain open to how your life might change when you learn to apply them with more flexibility and nuance in your life.

Questioning Hierarchy

Some Asian cultures, especially those influenced by Confucian values, view elder respect as one of the highest virtues. Within the community, there is often a strong hierarchy based on age, seniority, and knowledge. For many of us, the phrase "respect your elders" is deeply ingrained in our interactions with others. From a young age, I recall being expected to defer and not question those who were older. I often complied not out of respect for that particular person, who sometimes was a stranger, but out of respect and honor for my own parents. I was quite aware that my parents could be judged within our community by how well I followed these rules of social hierarchy.

And while this virtue is something I can still appreciate and value, I also have come to question this hierarchy framework and whether I might need to practice this virtue with much more flexibility than I was taught by my parents and culture. I can see how this compliance to hierarchy has kept me from questioning or challenging the status quo simply in an effort to be viewed as obedient, good, or nice.

It was this hierarchy mindset that kept me silent when a male supervisor repeatedly made me uncomfortable with his suggestive looks and comments about my appearance. For several years, I bit my tongue and showed up to work with dread. I was miserable. I was taught to allow those higher up in the hierarchy (i.e., older, male, white, higher status, more power) to dictate how they interact with me without protest or consequence. It took many years of questioning to finally realize that respecting my elders was something that did not have to be absolute; instead, I owed it to myself to decide when elders deserve my respect.

I have promised myself that I will not teach my children to comply with adults simply because they are older. I'll teach them how to evaluate whether an individual deserves their respect regardless of their age. I will not allow them to silence themselves simply because of seniority. I will not allow them to be bullied by those who might threaten to minimize their ideas or feelings simply because they are younger. I will teach them boundaries and encourage them to protect themselves.

REST STOP

I encourage you to question this hierarchy framework and wonder how you might have internalized these rules in your own life. Is it serving you? Is it helping you feel empowered or honest about your experiences? Or is it hindering or silencing you? We can offer respect and honor to older generations while also thinking critically of situations in which respecting our elders might be problematic.

Questioning Success and Scarcity Mindset

The only career choices for children of immigrants are doctor, lawyer, or engineer. We've all heard this joke, right? This is certainly not the case for all Asian parents, but it speaks to the strong value placed on financial stability and independence. Often, we come to value things we believe we lack most. A common experience for immigrant parents is the arrival in another country—the United States or elsewhere—in a state of scarcity or poverty. It makes sense that our parents adopted a scarcity mindset, believing that they would never have enough resources to feel stable and safe. While this mindset may have kept our parents working hard, sacrificing personal and mental health, and pushing through overwhelming struggles to establish themselves, this mindset may have also limited what they believed possible for their children and restricted their measures of success. If financial stability is the only goal for life, then money and wealth may be the only measures that count.

Unfortunately, these definitions of success may not align with our own. Instead, you might dream of creativity, service, advocacy, entrepreneurship, passion, alignment with talents, and careers that your parents may not have even realized, or currently realize, exist. The truth is that (most of) our parents love us and their drive for stability is intended to prevent us from having to struggle in the ways that they may have. For most of us, it is their intention of love that drives them to push certain career paths and goals. It is the safe path that they know.

As children of immigrants, questioning our parents' definitions of success may be one of the hardest spaces for us. For some of us, our definitions of success may align with our parents', in which case there is little friction. But for others, questioning their definitions of success may prompt major conflict within our relationships. In questioning their definitions of success, we may no longer conform to their expectations. We step off the well-marked path and possibly trigger anxiety and fear in them. We may feel like we have let our parents down or wasted all their hard work. We may be terrified to take risks and pursue our passions and dreams because the possibility of failure may feel catastrophic. We may also believe that success is linear and so any mistakes or failures can deeply injure our confidence and self-esteem. This rigid mindset, that success is narrowly defined by a certain income, position, or profession, means that anything short of that strict standard is viewed as failure. What an exhausting way to live.

⸺ **REST STOP** ⸺

Consider for a moment how your parents define success. What do they seem to value? Is it wealth, status, fame, stability, knowledge, service, creativity, entrepreneurship? How might you have internalized their values in your own pursuit of education or careers? Is there alignment between what you value and what your parents value? Finally, how would you define success in your own life?

Questioning Family Duty and Guilt

One of the strongest narratives for children of immigrants from many cultures is the story of our parents' sacrifice and suffering. In witnessing their struggle, many of us may believe that we need to somehow repay them by sacrificing parts of our own lives. It is difficult to think about my life without seeing family at the core. As the eldest daughter, I am used to looking out for and fulfilling different roles for my family of origin. Many children of immigrants can remember stepping into parental roles like negotiating the electric bill or translating at the doctor's office, due to language and cultural barriers. Our sense of responsibility for and duty toward our parents and family are ingrained at an early age. This sense of responsibility is not inherently bad—it is something that many might take pride in. Some may gladly welcome the opportunity to take care of their parents, while others might struggle beneath the weight of duty and wonder if they are able to carry it all. Many of us may also wonder where the line is between giving to others out of love and respect while also saving some of ourselves for our own needs and wants.

This tension between self and others is an ongoing growth process for children of Asian diasporas. We were simultaneously raised in two cultures: one that values independence and autonomy while the other encourages us to sacrifice and accommodate for family, as an act of love. It is such a confusing space to live in. It requires so much discernment and judgment to decide when to listen to our own wants and needs and when to honor others through our actions and decisions.

If we choose ourselves over family, we might also experience intense guilt. Guilt is such a prevalent emotion for children of immigrants and can drive so much decision-making. It can make us feel ashamed or regretful. It can cause us to bypass ourselves for the "greater" good. It can prevent us from communicating and establishing healthy boundaries with the people we love. This is why it is so important to question these family expectations and our possible feelings of guilt, because it is easier to ignore our own voice when the expectations or feelings of duty are strong. It is more efficient to play the role of the fixer, saver, and problem solver than to think critically about your capacity and boundaries. It is easier to do it yourself than to involve others, ask for help, or find alternative solutions. But at what cost? For how long? And how sustainable is it?

In truth, there have been many times in life when I chose others over myself simply to avoid complexity, believing that I was acting out of love, only to become resentful and stew about it for days. Other times, I induced so much internal guilt that I ignored my inner voice just so I could please others and be liked. It is easier to live in the binary space that is prioritizing others and denying the self than to negotiate the messiness of communicating my own needs and wants while staying connected to others. Consider the gray spaces, wherein you might find that self-sacrifice does not have to be the only way, and that loving people in your life also means you must learn how to love and value yourself.

⌣⌣⌣ R E S T   S T O P ⌣⌣⌣

How do you view yourself in relation to your family or family of origin (the family that you grew up with)? What expectations do you and they have about your role in their lives? Do you feel a tension between their needs and wants and your own? Be curious about that tension. Try not to ignore or suppress the feeling of push and pull. Give yourself permission to listen to your true wants and needs. What deep longing exists there?

Questioning Emotions and Vulnerability

Emotions are weak. You need to swallow them. Pretend they don't exist. Don't let it impact you otherwise you are weak. You are stronger than this. Just stop crying.

Do messages like these feel familiar? Received from our parents, families, or society overall, these messages convey that emotions are bad and disruptive. You need to shut them down. What's most damaging about these messages is that so few of us understand why we have emotions anymore. And even worse, so few of us understand how to decode emotions and use them to our benefit. Questioning how we relate to our emotions is a critical part of identity work. Think of your emotions as guideposts that help you decide whether you are on the right path. Your emotions encourage you to check in and ask yourself, "Does this feel right? What is this stirring up in me? Why am I feeling this way?" The problem is that many of us have actually learned to mistrust our emotions, believing that they might lead us astray.

As children of Asian immigrants, we may have been also

taught to save face, the cultural value of maintaining the positive impression or reputation of yourself and your family through your actions and deeds. We may have been taught that emotions, which show vulnerability, could cause us to lose face or create a negative impression of ourselves and our families. We may have been told to hide our emotions, family conflicts, and the messiness of our lives in secrecy and shame, which only further isolates and drives us into hiding the pain—all in an effort to preserve the façade that everything is okay.

As a new generation of Asian immigrants, we need to deeply question the cost of avoiding emotions and vulnerability in our lives. Many of us were never taught that emotions are actually neither good nor bad; they are vital to our survival. Without emotional vulnerability, we cut off authentic connection with others and lose out on the important knowledge that our emotions provide us. Far too many of us have been taught to ignore the emotional signs and push through despite what our minds and bodies are telling us, and then to label this self-denial as a sign of strength. If we continue to ignore, suppress, and disregard our emotional lives, we will struggle to move forward in understanding what we want and the life we want to live. We must actively challenge some of our instinctual responses of pushing our emotions aside in favor of staying in control.

⌒ REST STOP ⌒

How do you relate to your emotions? Can you identify them? Do you trust them? Do you listen to them? What are the narratives that keep you from listening to and expressing your emotions? What are the narratives that keep you from sharing them with trusted and safe people?

Questioning Indebtedness and Asking for Help

I remember watching my parents play an infuriating—yet comical—game when I was a child. Any act of kindness or gift giving prompted a sense of indebtedness. It was so strong that my parents felt compelled to return the act or gift with an even grander gesture. If someone had given us a gift of $100 in value, we had to "repay" them with a gift of at least $100 or greater. Does this scenario give you an idea of how complex the notion of asking for help might be within my family and culture? Perhaps it's that way in yours, too.

For a long time, I believed that being hyper-independent was a positive thing. It meant that I was capable, strong, and ready to handle anything that came my way. That was until I became a mother. When my daughter was an infant, I took a trip with her alone and ran out of baby wipes in the airport. Of course, there were no stores in the terminal that sold a single pack of baby wipes. I frantically walked all around the terminal with her in a soiled diaper trying to find some alternative that might work. It took everything in me to finally ask another mother for some wipes. I think I even offered to pay her for them. She graciously offered the entire package to me and told me just to keep them all, as she had packed extras. I walked away feeling a mixture of gratitude and shame.

A common barrier to asking for help from others is feeling like a burden or inconvenience to others, which has been framed as shameful or disrespectful. And beyond that, some of my clients have shared that they don't ask for help because it means that they will "owe" for the favor. This relational indebtedness is something many of us were told to avoid at all costs. In many ways, you might have been taught that relationships were transactional instead of abundant and generous. But what if there was a different way of being in relationship with others? What if people genuinely cared about you and wanted to help you with no strings attached? What if your inability to receive that help hurt no one else but you? These are the questions that surfaced as I tried to go it alone for so many years of my life.

Within my culture and in my parents' immigration journey, there is and was such a premium placed on being self-reliant and self-sufficient. The very idea of asking for help can stir up so much shame or guilt; for me, it was shame that I didn't have it together enough or was not prepared enough to handle all outcomes. Over the years, I have realized that I used my hyper-independence as a way to protect myself from judgment and to save face. It also allowed me to use my independence as a metric by which to judge others for not having their stuff together—to admittedly feel superior or better than others. To keep the façade going. I have had to deeply question what benefit I receive if I pretend that I can do it all on my own. I also have had to understand that my inability to ask for and receive help has kept me from deeper, more authentic relationships with others who seek to be in community with me. It has been such a rich but humbling and uncomfortable unlearning process.

⟋⟍ **R E S T   S T O P** ⟋⟍

Do you ask for help? Do you know how to receive help without guilt or shame? What keeps you from reaching out to trusted people for support? What is it costing you to live as if you were an island?

Questioning Invisibility and Humility

As an Asian American woman, I have been taught my entire life to exist in the margins. Succeed, but don't become too visible. Excel, but don't take up space. Blend in and assimilate. All of this will keep you safe. It has taken me thirty-eight years to finally say thank you after receiving a compliment. It is a small win, but it took years to achieve. There is something utterly uncomfortable about being recognized and praised. Being visible makes my skin crawl and my stomach tighten up. Perhaps this is where some of my recurrent imposter syndrome comes from: the feeling that if I am recognized, I might also be at risk of being exposed as a fraud.

When I was a child, being boastful was discouraged. One does not point out one's own accomplishments. We let our work speak for itself. My parents never spoke of my accomplishments in public, though many of their friends didn't seem to share this reluctance. In fact, there were times when my parents minimized my accomplishments as an act of humility. I can understand why they held back, believing that humility was a virtue and their restraint was a sign of maturity. However, I remember thinking that their unwillingness to share about my accomplishments perhaps meant that they also were not proud, that I was still not good enough and, in turn, perhaps I should not be proud of myself or acknowledge my accomplishments either.

There is something elusive about feeling deserving or good enough just because you exist. I always thought deservingness was something you painstakingly earned. I had not realized that some people went about their lives fully capable of taking up space even though they hadn't proven a single thing. This constant sense of needing to prove yourself and earn your place in this world can keep us in constant fear, especially as immigrants and people of color, who have been forced to live in the margins and only conditionally accepted. Assimilation is a survival tool. Our ability to stay under the radar means that at least we have less chance of being noticed and possibly attacked or targeted.

However, staying invisible and humble comes at a cost. Many Asian Americans struggle to self-promote at work or advocate for themselves when they believe they have earned recognition. Somehow the virtue of humility has not always translated as positive in Western culture. Instead, it can at times be viewed as a lack of confidence, assertiveness, or leadership ability. It may also have contributed to the perpetuation of Asian stereotypes, such as being compliant and docile. As a community, we also saw that our invisibility did little to protect us from the violence and racially motivated attacks on Asians after the COVID-19 pandemic began to spread worldwide. We must question whether this way of showing up in the world is still working for us. We must wonder whether remaining hidden truly helps us move toward our goals, and whether it brings us into an empowered or disempowered place as individuals and a community.

—— REST STOP ——

Do you feel uncomfortable when attention is focused on you and your accomplishments? Do you struggle to share about your wins, even if internally you are super excited about them? Does it feel wrong to share about accomplishments because it feels boastful? Gently explore those narratives and question these fears. Ask yourself how invisibility might be keeping you safe. Also wonder to yourself, what does your invisibility cost you?

FINDING YOUR COMPASS

The problem with living your life based on a map is that all the paths are already filled in for you. A map does not reflect your true reality. You assume that a certain route is going to work out for you because others have taken that path before you. Maybe it's your older sibling or your parents' friends' kids (whom they love to compare you with) who have all taken this road before, and they seem just fine. Except now you are on this path, and everything inside of you is filled with dread or ambivalence or both.

When we open the door and give ourselves permission to question, it can be quite unnerving. Suddenly, ideas and frameworks we assumed were working for us no longer seem to fit. This can trigger a lot of uncertainty; without other people's definitions of success or happiness to model after, where exactly do we go from here? Many clients—and I, myself—experience a mixture of thrill and freedom at the possibility, only to experience self-doubt and fear in the next second. This is completely normal and a sign that you are doing the difficult work of recalibrating your way of living and being. This means that you are starting to see new trailheads and paths emerge, ones that you have never noticed before.

Now that we have decided to toss the map out the window, where do we go from here? We begin by asking ourselves some more difficult questions:

- What do I value?
- What matters to me?
- What kind of person do I want to become?
- What things do I stand for?
- What am I willing to consistently show up for in my life?

- What would I do when no one is watching?
- What brings me joy?
- What brings me passion?
- What brings me purpose?

- What makes me feel safe?
- What excites me?
- What problem in this world could I uniquely solve?

This book could be filled with questions like this—though it would be an arduous process. So many people have revealed to me that once they are able to separate themselves from the expectations and aspirations of others, they actually have no idea what they want, because they have never been taught or encouraged to understand what they want. They have not practiced the muscle of self-introspection and discernment. They do not know how to listen to themselves.

If you are uncertain of where to start, I encourage you to begin with an exploration of your core values. Core values are what I like to call the cardinal signs of your life compass. They form the core of what you are working toward and the person you believe yourself to be. They are adaptable and evolving, but also stable and grounding. When you are faced with difficult decisions, returning to your core values reminds you of what you have chosen to focus on for this season of your life and keeps you on your desired course.

VALUES-BASED LIVING

Living in accordance with goals means to be focused on external outcomes and benchmarks: Finishing college. Getting a job. The next promotion. Getting married. It is a focus on a destination, whether that destination is a person, place, or thing. It has us focused on arriving at a place where we believe we will finally be happy or satisfied. Except many of us have been on this path before, and it turns into a treadmill that does not stop. Each time you achieve a goal, there is hardly time to celebrate, because you are already headed toward the next benchmark. With goals-based living, you ignore all the parts of yourself that do not directly help you reach that specific goal. You work long hours. You ignore important relationships. You keep making excuses instead of taking care of your mind and body. You just keep telling yourself to keep hustling because you can rest when you get your goal, except you never do.

In stark contrast, values-based living means living your life from a set of core values focused on the person you believe you are and the person you would like to become. It is much less concerned about the outcomes that are produced or achieved, but instead focuses on whether we are living true to the values that define who we are. Living from our values forms the internal compass that keeps us steady, even when everything in life hits the fan and threatens to pull us off course. Our core values shape our identity and help us build resiliency, because we work hard to define ourselves by guiding principles instead of outcomes that we often do not have control over. Without a sense of our core values, we are adrift and easily tempted or influenced by outside forces. You may not think you have core values, but you *do* have them; you just haven't identified them yet. Your behaviors, how you spend your time, and what you prioritize reflect your core values, whether you have defined them or not.

A Season of Illness

In 2019, my partner became ill. His symptoms were so subtle that at first we thought it was mild indigestion. As the year progressed, the pain worsened, and it became harder and harder for him to get through his day. Suddenly, we started talking about backup plans in case he could no longer work, and how we would support our family on a single income. Our young children, aware that something was wrong with Daddy, often asked us whether we could go back to the "normal days."

These next two years of our lives were some of the hardest I could imagine, as the COVID-19 pandemic shut everything down a month after he was hospitalized. Some days were so difficult that it took everything in my power to get up each morning and face my hopeful kids. Each day I struggled with the uncertainty of what was to come and the grief of all that we had lost in this season of illness. It was during this time that I had to strip myself back down to my core values. Daily meditation on these core values kept me afloat. For once, our future had no identifiable benchmarks. We had no idea what our future would look like. We could no longer set goals. We no longer made future plans because we could not predict when or how he might feel better.

Consistent exercise—I prefer running—and holding on to my core values saved me. Without those two things to focus on, I am not certain I could have survived. There were days when I would tell myself all I had to do was survive until dinnertime. If I could do that, then I would have succeeded for the day. In those hours before dinner, it was my core values that gave me purpose and also reminded me that if I burned myself out, the entire ship would sink with my children and partner inside.

Getting at Your Core Values

What exactly are core values? They are the highest values or beliefs that an individual or organization operates from. These core values are the cornerstones of how we make decisions, interact with others, and guide our behaviors. What is important to remember is that our core values can change over time, and in fact I try to revisit my core values yearly or even quarterly, especially if there are many things stressing me out and vying for my attention.

When my partner was ill, I had three core values:

1. Family
2. Making a difference
3. Well-being

My family had to be my priority because I had young children and could not reliably count on my partner for help, especially when he was feeling extremely ill. We also had limited family support because my partner's condition worsened right as the pandemic hit, and we could not risk getting our elderly parents sick.

It was during this time that I began my social media account @asiansformentalhealth, which was a space that allowed me to see some perspective and make a larger impact. Few of my followers knew that during the entire first few years of this account, I was going through one of the hardest seasons of my life. It was the shared stories and encouragement of this online community that gave me another focus when some days just felt too hopeless and hard.

And finally, I had to focus on keeping myself healthy in mind and body for the sake of my children and partner. There were days where I could feel the pull of hopelessness and depression because

I was so distraught over my partner's condition that it would make me want to hide under the covers and do nothing but watch Netflix all day. Instead, I would make sure that I was scheduled to see my therapist or go for a run the next day. It was difficult to stay connected with others during this time because of the pandemic and my partner's health, but part of maintaining my well-being was being honest and vulnerable with those who could receive me. I remember calling my best friend and just crying. At the end of the call, she said, "I don't know that you have ever been so vulnerable like this before." It was the truth. In our twenty-five years of friendship, I am not certain I had ever cried with her or anyone like I did that night.

It was through this extremely difficult season that I was slowly breaking down all of the rules and questioning all my previous ways of being. It hurt to go through this process, but in the course of the journey, it started to set me free. Doing this work helped me realize that these rules about how I should show up actually kept me stuck and very alone.

IDENTIFYING YOUR CORE VALUES

Let's start mapping out your core values. Please do not skip this step. Getting in touch with your core values is an important aspect of identity work.

Go to the appendix of this book (page 269) to find a list of core values. First, mark all the words that seem to resonate or create a stir in you. Then, go through the list again and try to narrow down your core values to three. Think about what you want to focus on during the next three to six months and which core values help remind you of this focus.

Once you have identified your three core values, list them below.

Core Value #1: _____

Core Value #2: _____

Core Value #3: _____

Now that you have identified your core values, start thinking about specific behaviors you might engage in that would align with these core values. Core values cannot just be held in thought. They must match our behaviors. For example, if one of my core values was well-being, but I frequently overworked myself, did not set boundaries, and often canceled my own personal therapy if I was too busy with work, then my behaviors would indicate a misalignment with that core value. When our behaviors reflect our core values, they self-reinforce that they are important to us—so important that we prioritize these behaviors or actions in the midst of all the things fighting for our attention. However, if these behaviors drop off, it might be an indication either that this core value is not as important as you thought or that you have some barriers to remove in order to align your behaviors with your core values.

To help you, here's how I mapped my core values:

Core Value #1: *Family*

1. Spend time with kids individually at least once per month
2. Have an intentional check-in with my partner once a week, even when we are exhausted
3. Stop working by five p.m. regardless of what is still left to do

Core Value #2: *Make a difference*

1. Focus on clinical care
2. Share a mental health post at least once a week
3. Work on developing the Asian American and Pacific Islander therapist directory

Core Value #3: _Well-being_

1. Running two or three times a week
2. Weekly therapy
3. Touch base with a close friend at least twice a month

What is helpful about living from core values is that it helps tune out the noise. As my social media account started to grow, there were more and more requests for my time and energy. I wanted to say yes to everything that this important work was bringing my way; however, I had to pause when these requests started to interfere with my other core values of family and well-being. As I started to participate in more and more events, it started impacting my ability to show up for my family and to protect my mental health. Over time, this misalignment started to reveal itself; as I became more stressed, I realized I had started to compromise my other core values in service of another. Growing anxiety and stress became clear signposts that something was no longer working. Recalibration had to happen in my actions and decisions in order to bring my life back into alignment. This is how core values keep us centered. They remind us of what is important when everything in life claims to be important. They also remind us that we are often living in the tension between spaces and that when we give ourselves permission to question that tension, we come to know more about ourselves.

*　　　*　　　*

As we close this chapter, my hope is that you can see how questioning is a necessary and vital first step of our identity work, as human beings and as members of Asian diasporas. There are many unique spaces in which we need to ponder, as we learn how to negotiate between the people we love, a world that views us in a certain light, and our own internal and emotional lives. I hope you accept my invitation to question all the frameworks you may have assumed were unchangeable and fixed. I hope that you are thinking deeply about your core values, as they will become your inner guide and keep you focused on what is most important. And finally, I hope you release yourself from the weight of having to know exactly how this turns out, because your journey is just beginning. I am excited for you to watch yourself slowly unfold.

CHAPTER 2

Permission to Feel

Control your emotions or they will control you.
—Chinese proverb

Imagine being in the midst of an emotional tidal wave. You can feel the surge of emotion cutting through your chest like a hot knife. Every atom in your body is trembling with so much kinetic energy that you have a hard time settling down. Now imagine being told in the midst of that emotional groundswell to stop. Just stop it. Forcibly swallow that burning lump of coal in your throat and shove it all down. Many children of immigrants, Asian and otherwise, may have received these messages throughout childhood. In Mandarin Chinese, there is even an expression for this emotional swallowing: 吃苦, the idea of "swallowing your bitterness" as a way to cope with strong emotions and hardships. Swallowing became a sign of strength, a sign of mastery over oneself, a sign of maturity. At least that is what I thought for most of my life.

Our early ideas about emotions are often shaped through our family of origin, which is a fancy way of saying the family you grew up in. My first experiences with emotions were kind of confusing. My mother was quite emotionally expressive. She has always said that any strong emotion could make her cry, be it joy, sorrow, or anger. But even with this openness to expressing emotion, she struggled to trust and listen to her emotions in the midst of the hierarchical and patriarchal systems that pushed back against her within her marriage and community. While she could express her emotion through tears, the tears were usually where it ended. She usually ended up brushing her emotional upset aside and labeled herself as too sensitive or emotional in hindsight.

I can clearly recall my mother breaking down in tears from the overwhelming stress of being a young immigrant mother. Sometimes these tears were due to homesickness. Other times it was anger at how American society viewed her. Many times, her tears were the result of the cultural and generational gaps that we could not seem to bridge in our relationship. These gaps caused so much conflict during my teenage years that I continue to feel much regret and sorrow over the tears she shed during that season of my life. My only solace is the thought that we were on the journey of learning: learning how to be with each other in emotion, how to express that emotion, and how to use that emotion to deepen our relationship. But my goodness, was it messy and painful during the many lessons of that journey.

My father, on the other hand, was silent and stoic. Occasionally, his anger or irritation would spill over into our interactions, creating a sense of disappointment and self-blame that has taken me a lifetime to work through and heal from. In my teenage years, we fought relentlessly because I refused to yield to his expectations of hierarchy and authority. In those moments, I was not certain our relationship could ever recover. During those conflicts, my strong emotions only further cemented his belief that I was "too emotional," lacking in rationality and logic, which gave him more reason to stonewall me when I would not give in. Looking back, I realize it was our mutual lack of emotional literacy and poor communication skills that caused us so much strife.

It was between these two spaces that I started to piece together how and what I was allowed to feel as a young Asian American woman. I learned that people interpreted my emotions based on my gender. Women who were willing to express emotion were viewed as weak, lacking in control, or too sensitive, while men capable of suppressing emotion were viewed as strong, psychologically tough, and more rational. My own parents seemed to reflect this sexist narrative, and I naïvely assumed that these emotional caricatures were true. I struggled to understand how emotions could be useful or helpful in my life. Instead, emotions felt like they were more effort than they were worth. They were time-consuming, messy, upending, and difficult. It has taken me a lifetime to break down these patriarchal, sexist, and harmful narratives so I can freely embrace my emotions with awareness and compassion, and, even more important, to realize that my emotions are vital tools that will guide me along my journey back home to myself.

Many clients and individuals within Asian diasporas have shared that emotions are viewed by the outside world as not valid, not valued, not welcome, not normal, and not to be trusted. They have been told that emotions are meant to be sucked up, suppressed, overridden, controlled, distrusted, and held back to make others more comfortable. So many of us have come to believe that emotions are threatening, useless, and unworthy of our attention—if only we could just make our negative emotions go away. The story sold to us has been that emotions are the threat and should be extinguished. We also have been told that emotions make others uncomfortable, and so we must silence our emotions as an act of self and communal preservation. But if emotions are so bad for us, then why are they still around? Why have emotions been preserved across human evolution if they are pointless for our psychological lives? Wouldn't life be better if we didn't experience emotional highs and lows and just stayed even-keeled every day? These are the questions we must explore.

In this chapter, I extend a second invitation to you—to give yourself the permission to feel and embrace your emotions as a vital part of living a healthy life. I believe that if we do not allow ourselves to feel and experience our emotions, we carry forward many painful parts of ourselves like open wounds that refuse to heal. Changing how we relate to our emotions also gives us the ability to break intergenerational cycles of trauma and pain that our parents may have unknowingly passed along to us. We must feel in order to heal those parts of ourselves.

We also must explore how our various cultures may have inadvertently encouraged us to ignore and suppress our emotions, as a trauma-based coping strategy. We will discuss how our parents, with their emotional and psychological blind spots, may not have had the tools and skills to help us accept and embrace our emotions as valid, necessary, and critical. We offer no blame or judgment for their inability to teach us skills that they themselves lacked, but only compassion for how difficult it must have been to hold space for our emotions in the midst of their own emotional valleys, as immigrants to new countries.

REST STOP

How do you relate to your emotions? What are the voices that emerge when you experience emotions? Are they kind, tender, and nurturing, or are they harsh, critical, and judging? Where do you think those voices came from? How would you like to relate to your emotions instead?

BARRIERS TO EMOTIONAL ACCEPTANCE

Several barriers keep us, as children of Asian immigrants, from learning the necessary skills to relate to our emotions in more effective and positive ways. Some of them are cultural, while others are impacted by various narratives and stereotypes that have been placed on us and people who look like us. Our parents, in their best efforts to equip us for this world, may have tried to shield us in the best ways that they knew, which was to teach us how to harden ourselves to the ups and downs of emotions. As immigrants with limited language abilities, it may have been easier to shut down emotional responses in order to show up for work and deal with a racist boss or to push through the grief and sadness of losing a parent halfway across the world and not having the money to travel home to attend their funeral. The suppression of emotion may have been the most effective tool that they had in their emotional tool kit, which is why they passed it along to you and me.

Emotional avoidance, as a short-term strategy, can sometimes give us space to calm down our bodies and nervous systems. It might also allow us to temporarily step back from overwhelming triggers in order to respond more intentionally. However, some of us may start to overrely on avoiding negative emotions as a long-term strategy, which quickly becomes problematic. Sometimes we think that if we just keep avoiding the negative emotion, then we won't need to actually face the cause of that negative emotion; we won't need to actually acknowledge and listen to what this emotion might be telling us. It also keeps us from having to make hard decisions or accept hard truths about our lives. It is this overreliance on emotional avoidance that can stand in the way of us being able to harness our emotions and use them to our benefit.

In fact, simply avoiding negative emotions doesn't make them go away; it only pushes them deeper inside, where they fester like an infected wound. When we drive these emotions underground, they start to pollute our emotional water system, which wreaks havoc on all parts of our psychological and physical health. While this avoidance strategy starts off as self-protection, it is a costly strategy, because it causes us to mistrust our emotions and locks us out from the deep knowledge that our emotions reveal to us about our lives.

For many of our parents, emotional suppression may have meant survival. Emotional suppression may have allowed our parents to stay safe from abusive or toxic parents who took out their rage on them. For others, emotional suppression protected them from dangerous political regimes that conquered their homelands and imprisoned any dissenters or activists. These historical contexts, sometimes left out of our family narratives due to trauma, may explain why our parents passed down the coping skill of ignoring or suppressing our emotions. My mother once explained she was taught that strong emotionality, either positive or negative, was seen as potentially harmful to the physical body, which is why the expression of strong emotions was discouraged. Thankfully, our generation is starting to change these narratives around mental health. We are realizing that our mental health is something that must be protected and prioritized. We are starting to challenge and question these intergenerational and cultural frameworks about emotions because they might not be serving us well any longer. If we don't challenge these frameworks, we run the risk of passing down the same coping mechanisms to our children, which will not serve them in their unique life context either.

Emotions give us the motivation and energy to enact change in our lives and to decide that we no longer want to stay the same because we are so sick and tired of the same dynamics, same problems, and same feeling of dissatisfaction with our lives. Emotions can light a fire beneath us and move us forward in our growth. Making this change also helps us realize that we are no longer living in alignment with our core values and that we need to do something about it. Before we get there, let's explore some barriers to emotional acceptance for children of Asian immigrants.

Saving Face and Stoicism

As mentioned in chapter 1, the cultural value of saving face is a powerful one. It creates a sense of deep responsibility over how we show up in our world and highly values how the world in turn sees us. It also ropes in the emotion of shame when we fail to uphold the images that we are expected to project. Most people think of this as the need to avoid public embarrassment or shame due to one's actions, behaviors, and appearances. But there is much more to it than that. The "face" is also a public persona or value on which we ascribe positive and negative properties. It is a reflection of not only the individual but also the persona of the family and communities that each individual represents. Maintaining your "face" may look like obtaining a well-paying job and making sure your life seems perfect, which enhances the "face" of our families as well. We may "lose face" when we are involved in a situation or behavior that goes against social norms or societal expectations and, as a result, brings down the face of our entire family as well. Perhaps you have been told your entire life that it is your job to maintain that familial "face," even if it means denying parts of yourself. Talk about pressure!

If one of your cultural values is saving face, then the idea of revealing your intimate emotions becomes deeply uncomfortable, even with trusted and loving people. Revealing how we feel about our family flaws, conflicts, or problems can be viewed as being disloyal to our family. This code of privacy surrounding family life is one of the reasons why we might be hesitant to seek support from others or even reach out for professional mental health help, because the act of being vulnerable and honest about our emotions and struggles can be seen as exposing our family secrets and bringing shame upon ourselves and our families. Notice how this cultural value impacts not only how we engage with others, but also whether we can even give ourselves permission to feel our negative emotions without judgment and criticism.

——— **REST STOP** ———

Can you imagine how you might relate to your emotions if one of your cultural values was vulnerability instead of saving face? What if our culture prioritized spaces and relationships that allow us to be honest, raw, and real with each other? How would that change how you show up with your emotions? What would you do differently if you could just be real and not have to maintain a face?

Comparing Our Suffering to Our Parents' Suffering

As children of immigrants, the idea that our parents suffered far more than we ever could have or will may make it quite difficult for us to express negative emotions or unhappiness about our lives. In light of our parents' suffering, we may feel ashamed or guilty that we are complaining about our own lives, even if we are deeply unhappy. The narrative that the one who suffers the most hardship is the only one allowed to express frustration has caused many of us to silence our feelings of depression, anxiety, sadness, or discontent. How can I complain about my life if I have a stable income from a job that allows me to sit inside an office and drink a latte each morning while my parents stood for hours in convenience stores and laundromats or worked as manual laborers or domestic workers just trying to make ends meet? Giving ourselves permission to feel in the backdrop of these stories and narratives can prompt such strong feelings of guilt that it might be easier to deny how we feel.

However, let's wonder for a moment. How does denying your own experience change your parents' history or experiences? How does ignoring your own feelings of frustration or discontent somehow repay them for their suffering? The reality is that it cannot. Our denial of our emotional experiences has no tangible impact on our parents' past histories. However, our focus on the comparative suffering between ourselves and our parents does have the possibility of negatively impacting our own lives and future goals. Our unwillingness to listen to our emotions might lead us to stay in an unfulfilling relationship. Ignoring our emotions might keep us stuck in situations that we know make us deeply unhappy. Instead, we could hold space for both/and. It can be true *both* that our parents struggled *and* that we can also struggle in our own unique ways. Both of our stories are valid, can be acknowledged, and met with empathy and compassion.

I believe that we need to reframe the notion that listening and expressing our negative emotion is an act of complaining and being ungrateful. Instead, listening to our negative emotions cues us to potential areas of growth and change. Our negative emotions uncover parts of our lives that are no longer working as they should and areas in our lives that we may need to shed in order to help us move forward. Instead of seeing negative emotions as representations of our selfishness or privilege, perhaps emotions are the necessary guideposts that help us realize if we have lost our way.

———— **R E S T   S T O P** ————

Do you find yourself avoiding your negative emotions because they trigger a sense of guilt? Do you compare your life to that of your parents and feel bad that you are not as grateful as you "should" be? Can you give yourself permission to feel the feelings of discontent and even admit that perhaps you aren't happy? Can you give yourself permission to realize that your unhappiness does not diminish or negate your parents' sacrifices, but instead might be the very privilege that they worked so hard for you to experience, the privilege of acknowledging your emotions and prioritizing your mental health?

Relational Harmony and Peacekeeping

How many times have you been encouraged to give up on your wants and needs simply because relationship harmony was prioritized over conflict? Perhaps you witnessed this play out between your parents, as their conflicts often resulted in one person repeatedly giving in and silencing themself in order to keep the peace. Or you were asked to give in to older or younger siblings simply because of their age and let go of your opinions or boundaries to keep the peace. Many of us may have subconsciously learned that we are responsible for protecting the emotions of our family members. Sacrifice for the common good is what they often told us; our choices and decisions should not incite conflict or create relational discord because peace allegedly matters more than our individual happiness.

While there is nothing inherently wrong with keeping the peace between family members, the emphasis on peace and harmony might send the implicit message that conflict is bad and should be avoided at all costs, even if it means that we need to emotionally bypass ourselves in order to maintain that peace. When we ignore our emotions, it is much easier to keep the peace and keep everyone calm and happy. Unfortunately, when peace is prioritized over conflict, we lose opportunities to build skills for communication, negotiation, and collaboration. So many of my Asian American clients struggle deeply with interpersonal conflict. It is something they try so hard to avoid that they learn to completely silence their emotions to avoid all conflict. When you are angry and aware of that anger, it is hard to stay silent and keep the peace. When you realize that you are not getting your needs met, you might need to speak up, and this might stir up conflict with others or make them upset. Instead of wading through the murky emotional waters that naturally rise within interpersonal relationships, sometimes we take what we believe to be the easier path, which is to shut down our emotions to maintain the peace.

However, one of the most important lessons we must learn is that we cannot control, change, or be responsible for the emotions of others. Repeat that to yourself *out loud*. Our emotions are entirely our own. We are each responsible for our own emotions and how these emotions cause us to act. While we can support and be with each other in our emotions, we cannot take other people's emotions on as our responsibility to fix, regulate, or tame. When someone becomes angry with you, it is not your job to make them feel better; it is their job to learn the skills to hold space for that anger and make themselves feel better. It is also their responsibility to understand their anger and, if necessary, communicate with you about how you might have contributed to that emotion within them. The problem is that so many of us have been on the receiving end of trouble from people who are totally clueless about how to take ownership over their own emotions. And what happens when people don't know how to own and manage their emotions? They project their negative emotions on us and make us believe that we caused the negative emotion. They make us believe that their negative emotions are our fault and problem to fix.

So many of us have learned about emotions through unspoken interactions. One of the most frustrating aspects of Asian culture is that important things are rarely said plainly or directly. This causes us to guess and assume one another's thoughts or feelings, and these guesses often miss the mark. This is why it is so important for us to develop the necessary skills to understand our emotions and express them more effectively, so we can finally set down the rudimentary survival tactics of peacekeeping, people pleasing, and emotional projecting.

―――― **R E S T　S T O P** ――――

Do you find yourself in the role of the peacekeeper in your relationships? How does staying in this role protect and benefit you? What does staying in this role cost you? Do you silence your emotions in order to maintain harmony within your relationships?

WHY BOTHER WITH EMOTIONS?

Emotions are a part of our lives as human beings, whether we want them to be or not. Emotions are a combination of our subjective experiences, physical sensations, and behaviors or reactions. When something happens to you that causes you to experience anger, the body and mind set off a cascade of hormones that impact your real-time experience. This emotional cascade is a hardwired part of our biology and evolution. In fact, without emotions we are much less likely to survive. We would not be prepared for possible threats. We would struggle to emotionally connect with our community, which offers us protection and connection. To put it simply, emotions are an alert system and give us information about ourselves and our environment.

If emotions provide us with information, then they aren't necessarily good or bad. They just are. For example, if you received a text message that there was a hurricane headed to your city, you wouldn't think to yourself that the text message itself was bad. The text message was simply the alert that something dangerous is or might be on the way. We tend to think emotions in and of themselves are the problem because of how upending and out of control they can make us feel in the moment. But if we can stay curious with our emotions long enough, we might actually be able to see through the chaos and understand the alert message hidden within them.

Clients often come to therapy thinking that if they work hard enough, they will be able to reduce or eliminate their negative emotions. They think that somehow they will find a way to no longer react to or get triggered by certain situations or people. In some situations, it might be possible to change how we interpret or appraise these triggering situations, which then can reduce the emotional upset that we experience, but the ultimate goal is not to make our emotions disappear, but rather to move through our emotions more effectively and to decode and understand the information that our emotions might be sending us.

Emotional Impact and Functionality

As much as we believe that we are logical and rational human beings, you would be surprised to realize how much of our lives is impacted by our emotions. Emotions have been found to impact how you see your world, what you pay attention to, what you learn and remember, and even how you make decisions. Western society seems to believe that making decisions from the rational mind instead of the emotional mind correlates with better outcomes. However, current research actually suggests that emotions are a crucial piece of overall decision-making, as people who experience damage to the emotional centers of the brain actually have problems making good decisions.

Whether you realize it or not, your emotions are activated throughout your day, and one of their primary functions is to protect you and make you self-aware. Negative emotions such as anger, irritation, frustration, and sadness direct the focus of your attention, pulling your awareness to the emotion rather than allowing you to go about your day as if everything was just fine. In fact, negative emotions tend to return if we fail to understand what is causing them and instead try to ignore or suppress them. Our emotions are alarms that say, "No, you are not fine! There is something you need to pay attention to!" Except many of us have hit the snooze button too many times, only to realize that the emotions return—and sometimes even louder. We must begin to realize that our emotions are guideposts that light our way in this confusing journey of life. And until we allow ourselves to stop hitting the emotional snooze button, we will never be able to harness the power of our emotions.

If the first function of emotions is to alert you and create self-awareness, then the second function is to help you communicate with others. Our species has survived precisely because we learned how to live in community. Many of our emotional survival instincts evolved so that we can quickly and easily communicate with each other. When we are insulted, for example, our bodies and minds react quickly and make a facial expression to communicate to the other person that we are upset even before we realize that our body language has given away our internal emotion. It is through these emotionally driven encounters that we can more efficiently read each other and anticipate the behaviors of others, all of which help us interact with each other more effectively. Beyond nonverbal communication, our emotions cue us to verbally communicate with one another if there is something misaligned in that relationship. Our emotions can help us form deeper bonds and relationships for survival through expressions of sympathy, empathy, compassion, forgiveness, and love. On the other hand, our emotions can also harm or damage relationships if they are poorly regulated and if we do not understand our emotions well enough to communicate with clarity what we need from each other.

Our emotions also have the ability to motivate us for action. When we experience an emotion, it triggers a cascade of bodily reactions that can have a lot of physical power. It also highlights the emotional importance (known as emotional salience) of this event, situation, and emotion. It helps us start to plan or organize for future action to address the situation that caused the emotion, or it helps us act in the moment. When a car is about to hit you on the freeway, your fear response activates you to swerve out of the way almost instantaneously. When you are upset that you were yet again overlooked for a promotion, this frustration and anger may prompt you to start actively looking for other jobs or planning a conversation with your boss in order to address your career progress. Emotions can stir up the emotional power and motivation you need to act in alignment with your core values and goals.

A Note on Emotional Sensitivity and Neurodiversity

While all humans experience emotions, we may experience our emotions differently. We can have different so-called emotional skins or emotional sensitivities. Some of us have thicker emotional skin due to a combination of genetics and life experiences, and may be less fazed by strong emotionality, while others have thinner skin and may feel seriously impacted by strong emotions within themselves or others. However, having thicker or thinner emotional skin is not inherently better or worse. There are some situations where having thicker or thinner skin might offer certain benefits or disadvantages. For example, I believe that because I'm a psychologist, my awareness of emotional experiences in myself and others helps me immensely in my therapeutic work with clients. This thinner skin means that I may be more aware and impacted by the emotions of others, which in this context is a strength. However, there might be instances in which this emotional sensitivity makes me more easily upset or triggered by others as well. We all approach life situations with different levels of sensitivity to emotions, and learning how to accept and work with your level of sensitivity is where the magic happens.

It is important to mention here that in addition to having different emotional skin, humans have a wide range of biological diversity. The term "neurodiversity" was coined by Judy Singer, a sociologist who studied the autism spectrum. Neurodiversity reflects the idea that humans have a wide range of ways we think, learn, and engage in our world, and that these are natural variations that should not be considered abnormal or a deficit. While an exploration of neurodiversity is beyond the scope of this book, there is certainly evidence that individuals experience emotions along a continuous spectrum and may express emotions in unique ways as well.

———— REST STOP ————

When you think about your emotions, can you wonder curiously about the functions of certain emotions in your life? How do these emotions protect, inform, and guide you? How do they lead you to take certain actions or explore different options? How might you approach your emotions with curiosity instead of judgment or mistrust?

BUILDING EMOTIONAL LITERACY SKILLS

I recently asked a question on social media: "What do you wish your parents or elders had taught you about your emotions when you were younger?" Some responses:

1. That it is okay to cry.
2. That it's okay to have emotions. It's normal and valid to give them space.

3. How to listen to and process emotions rather than just repressing.

4. How to express and discuss emotions and not bottle them up.

5. That emotions aren't a sign of weakness or something that you need to suppress.

I received hundreds of responses that reflected at least one of these five areas. In truth, we as a culture have done a poor job at equipping children, teens, and adults with emotional skills. These are skills we should be sharing in schools, workplaces, homes, and communities. Emotional literacy is simply the ability to understand and decode your emotions. And just like every other skill in your tool kit, it is something that can be learned and practiced.

When I first learned about emotions in graduate school, it felt so awkward. I had to ask, "What do you mean by 'listen to your emotions'?" I thought emotions were disruptive, damaging, distracting, and bad. Weren't they meant to be ignored and swallowed so deep that you could try to forget them? It has taken more than thirty-eight years to unlearn these messages, and even now that I am a psychologist, I still sometimes find myself distracting from my emotions with busyness and productivity, because emotions take time, and who has time these days! My therapist likes to joke, "If only awareness was enough to create lasting change." Being aware of how important our emotions are does not always translate into the discipline and practice of listening and patiently exploring our emotional lives. Here, I offer you some ways to begin this important practice and encourage you to adjust and tweak it with language and imagery that works for you.

Pause and Listen

As I reflect on my own upbringing, I realize that my mother had already started teaching me about these skills before I could put words to them. She likely didn't even have conscious awareness or knowledge that she was modeling emotion regulation skills. My first heartache occurred when I was a sophomore in college. I had ended a relationship that I thought was going to be lifelong. In truth, I probably knew for a few years that this was not the right relationship for me, but I held on because of the idealized image of a first love. After the breakup, I drove from Austin, where I was attending university, back to my parents' home in Houston for the weekend. I drove most of the three hours in tears, not sure how to fix the massive hole in myself. One night as I packed away all the pictures and mementos of that relationship, my mother simply held me as I sobbed. She did not curse this person for hurting me. She did not offer me any quick fixes to bypass the pain. She held me and sat with me for what felt like hours. She let me feel every sensation of heartbreak without distraction or dismissal. This is the first step in beginning to understand our emotions—just creating space to be *with* them. A moment in time for the emotion to exist without pushing it away or distracting us from it. Just pause and listen.

As children of immigrants, we may not have experienced what it felt like to pause and listen. Our parents might have been too overwhelmed. They might have been working long hours and too emotionally spent when they came home. They might have believed that focusing on negative emotions was harmful to your health and so encouraged you to suppress them. We were told "just stop crying," so instead of pausing and trying to listen to our emotions, we may have just pushed through, got busy, or found some easy distraction to skip over this step. But instead, what if when you felt strongly and deeply, you turned inward and paused? What if you held yourself like my mother held me? With stability, but tenderness. Without bypassing, shaming, or judgment. Step 1: Pause and listen.

Tolerate and Hold

In my work with clients—and sometimes even with myself and my kids—I sometimes use an exercise called the fishbowl. When I notice a strong emotion, I pause and imagine holding a round glass fishbowl. I then envision myself placing that intense emotion into this fishbowl, and I try to think about the colors, textures, and movement of this emotion as it swirls around inside. The goal here is to relate to your emotion with acceptance and awareness. The fishbowl allows you to focus and be aware of your emotion without being fused or stuck with your emotion, believing that it is all that you are capable of feeling or that this feeling will last forever. The thing with emotions is that they all eventually pass. They are fleeting and momentary compared to the overall length of our lives. Yet the surge of emotion comes like a wave, threatening to overcome us. But if we simply hold it and breathe through it, the surge eventually dies down. The struggle is that often these emotions can feel so intense and confusing that we feel like we are inside the fishbowl trying to escape as the emotion threatens to drown us.

My mother's presence that night, while I sobbed over my ex, functioned like a fishbowl. She held me in the moment, so I didn't have to stand there holding my pain alone. Her presence did not lessen my pain, but she held the pain with me and grounded me in a way that helped me realize that the pain would not destroy me, despite how painful it was in the moment. She demonstrated an idea called containment, even without her knowledge. Therapists use containment in practice to help hold space for clients in their emotions and experiences. The skill of tolerating and holding emotion is something that takes practice and time. As you practice, you build emotional tolerance and are able to expand your capacity for holding many different experiences without avoidance or running away. With consistent effort, you slowly teach yourself that emotions will not destroy you, that you are capable of holding them, and that they eventually pass through.

Some tips for practicing the fishbowl technique:

1. Let the emotion be. Let it exist.
2. Accept rather than resist. Allow the emotion to move within and through you instead of fighting against it.
3. Emotions are fleeting. You will not always feel this way.
4. If you are too overwhelmed, step back and breathe. Focus on how your body feels. Tune into your senses. What do you see, hear, taste, touch, and smell? You can always return to this emotion later. No need to push yourself into spaces that feel overwhelming or intolerable.

Notice and Understand

Negative emotions often prompt us to narrow the focus of our attention. When we are angry, we become pinpoint focused on thoughts and feelings related to our anger, and it can be hard to see other perspectives. It can make us fixate on the anger-inducing situation, chewing on it over and over. However, to be fully able to explore and understand our negative emotions, we need to be able to create some space. We need to be able to calm our nervous system and remind ourselves that we are not in immediate danger or under threat. When we are able to move away from a state of fight or flight, then we are able to expand our perspective and reasoning and begin to understand our emotions. It's why so many emotion regulation techniques emphasize some sort of breathing or mindfulness.

Deep breathing works to calm the nervous system, which reduces the fight-or-flight response. And when we engage in mindfulness, I am not talking about practicing a one-hour meditation session in the middle of your raging anger. Instead, mindfulness is simply the act of noticing. Notice how the body feels when you are scared. Notice the self-talk that you engage in when you are ashamed. Notice what is happening at that moment.

Even though we love each other deeply, my dad is one of my biggest triggers. He recently said to me, "You shouldn't let your nanny watch your kids so much. They are like cows grazing in the pasture." This is a Taiwanese expression, used to describe a person who is careless with the supervision or instruction of children. This comment struck me in the gut. When my partner got sick, I had to work more in order to help support our family, and there were real sacrifices in the process. His comment failed to acknowledge the efforts I was making to support our family through a difficult time. It also reflected his traditional perspectives about a woman's role as a mother. It took all my power not to lash out at him. Instead, I worked hard to notice what was happening in my body, as my stomach seized up and my heart rate increased. I reminded myself to breathe through my anger, focusing on the air entering my lungs and leaving through my nostrils. All this was an effort to calm my activated nervous system, which was screaming "What the hell?!" inside.

When I finally calmed myself down, I was able to see that my father was not trying to hurt me. He was concerned about my children and my well-being. His comment showed his love for my children and his concern about my overworking myself and harming my own health in the process. How he conveyed this concern was hurtful as hell, as his communication skills have always been somewhat lacking, but the intention behind his statement was not deliberately malicious. However, I would have never been able to see this situation with nuance and granularity without taking time to notice. And in noticing, I also was able to understand why this statement hurt me so much and consider how to communicate the impact of this hurtful statement to him, which leads us to our last and final skill.

Express and Take Action

There will be times when you pause and listen, tolerate and hold, notice and understand, and then decide that you may have learned something new about yourself or someone else but there is no action that you need to take. And this is totally okay. Not all emotions will lead to tangible action in the moment. It may just have been information that you are adding to your arsenal of knowledge about your life. But there will be other times, after you have walked through all of these steps, when you realize that you need to do something. It may be that you need to have a hard conversation or that you need to develop an action plan to make changes in your life.

Being able to express emotion is the transformation of inner knowledge and emotional knowing into verbal communication to share your emotional experience. Part of learning how to express our emotions is first learning the words to accurately describe how we feel. There are tools such as emotion wheels or mood meters available online that offer many different emotion-based words. We feel way more emotions than previously thought, and finding the words to describe them is the first step of expressing these emotions. For some of us, this may involve translating the emotion words into our mother tongue in order to express them to our parents.

When my father made that hurtful statement, I knew something had to be said, because otherwise he may not ever realize that the statement was hurtful, and I would implicitly be communicating that it was okay for him to say hurtful things to me. If I failed to communicate my emotional reaction to his statement, I would open up the possibility that he could do it again. I knew that my initial emotion was anger, followed by sadness and disappointment once I had calmed down. These emotions were showing me that this interaction was not okay and that I did not want to be in this same situation again. But how does one say this to someone who is not really great with emotions or communication? Knowing my own father, I think his defensive mechanisms are quite strong. If you come out swinging, he easily shuts down or plays things off as a joke. I had to approach with sincerity and firmness to convey that I was serious that he had hurt me.

When I need to offer feedback, I use two tools: "I" statements, and intention versus impact. "I" statements involve expressing thoughts and feelings from statements that begin with "I," for example, "Hey, Dad, I wanted to talk to you about something you said the other day. I felt really hurt when you said that my kids were like cows grazing in the pasture." This statement can be better received than a statement that begins with "you," which can come across as more accusatory or threatening: "You shouldn't have said that my kids were like cows grazing in the pasture. It really hurt me."

The intention versus impact tool can also be quite helpful in reducing defensiveness when expressing our emotions. I might have said, "Hey, Dad, you may not have intended to hurt me when you said that my kids were like cows grazing in the pasture, but those words impacted me in a hurtful way." Notice how we can name that one's intentions may not have been to do harm, while also acknowledging that the behavior was harmful and keep their behaviors accountable.

Another lesson I have had to learn in order to communicate my emotions, especially to my father, is that I cannot try to control his reaction or expect him to respond in a certain way, even after I have expressed my emotions or thoughts. If I expect a certain behavior from him, such as apologizing (which he has never done before), I set myself up for more anger and pain. But if my expectation is simply to communicate my emotions and experience so that he will know, in no uncertain terms, that his behavior or words were hurtful, then I am able to move forward toward forgiveness, *regardless* of his response. This may be a painful lesson for children of Asian diasporas, as the parent-child hierarchy can result in our parents never being willing to apologize or admit fault.

Some of us might think, *What is the point then of expressing our emotions or communicating about our conflicts if our parents won't ever apologize or admit that they messed up?* To that, I ask, "What do you have to gain by not communicating the impact of their actions and maintaining the same dynamic over and over?" Even if our parents never apologize or admit that they have harmed us, they now know which of their behaviors do harm. And while we cannot expect that they will ever change, when we express our emotions and take action rather than hide our emotions, we have now laid the foundation for future reminders to be communicated, which increases the chance that their behaviors might shift.

If your emotions have prompted you to take action, then this is when you get to the fun part. You get to create an action plan and start to work toward change in your life. Perhaps there is a tangible goal you would like to achieve or a core value you want to prioritize. Action plans require, well, action, and writing a list of actionable steps becomes one of the most concrete ways that you can measure your progress and hold yourself accountable to changes that you are making in your life. My favorite tip: Write down three actions that you are committing to and tape them to the bathroom mirror or another place you look every day. The daily reminder of these actions will increase your chances of completing them.

BREAKING DOWN YOUR EMOTIONS

This exercise is meant to help you deconstruct emotionally triggering situations based on the skills I shared with you in this chapter. Try to go through each part and, in your notebook, write your triggering event and phrases or thoughts for each section. Sometimes, you will be able to practice these skills in real time. Other times, you might do this after the fact, once the strong emotion has passed. I like to call these emotional excavations because they give us a chance to dig through what happened, what we felt, how we responded, and how we might behave differently the next time.

Triggering Event: _____

Pause and Listen: _____

What strategies did you use to remind yourself to pause? What worked? What didn't? What could you do next time to help you pause and listen?

Tolerate and Hold: _____

Did you feel the urge to skip, bypass, or ignore your emotion? How did you remind yourself to stay with and hold the emotion with tenderness? Were you able to hold your emotion in a vessel or fishbowl? Could you walk around the fishbowl with intention and focus?

Notice and Understand: _____

What did you notice, observe, and experience when watching the fishbowl? What did you notice in your body? What did you notice in your thoughts and self-talk? What did you notice about your feelings? What were your emotions trying to tell you? If they were trying to protect you, what might they be trying to protect you from?

Express and Take Action: _____

Did your emotions help you identify any conversations that might need to happen? Did your emotions highlight an area of your life that you might need to take action on? What would be the goal of these actions? Do these conversations or actions align with your core values?

Review: _____

Look back over this situation. How did it go? What are you proud of in how you showed up with your emotions this time? What might you do differently next time?

PERMISSION TO CRY

This may seem so simple, but it is important enough for me to dedicate an entire section to it. Crying is not just a way that we express our emotion; it is a biological function that allows us to process stress out of the body. It is a release we often need when we are overwhelmed, scared, or heartbroken. Crying is a part of the language of the body, and it can offer healing in ways that words struggle to do. For some of us, crying can feel vulnerable and unnatural. It may be something we choose to do alone or would prefer to do with safe people in our lives. It may take time for you to become comfortable with crying, and this is completely normal. We have to literally unwrap ourselves from the harsh narratives that we may have learned about what it means to cry. Be tender with yourself. And if all else fails, do what I do when I know I need to cry, but just cannot get myself to do it spontaneously: I put on a really sad movie and just let it all flow.

*   *   *

As we end this chapter, I hope you understand why it might be so difficult for you to navigate emotional spaces in your life. It is not your fault. It is simply because you did not know and did not have opportunity to practice. But now you know, and now you can practice. And in your deep emotional knowing, you now have the power to harness your emotions and break cycles of unknowing and swallowing for not only yourself, but also for generations that follow. When we give ourselves permission to feel, we are learning how to read our internal compass with more clarity and accuracy. Without our emotions, we live from places of "I should" or "they want me to" instead of turning inward for answers about what is right for our lives. And while I encourage you to be open to wise mentors and trusted people as you navigate your life, ultimately only you know what creates excitement, stirs passion, and brings you peace. All of your emotions exist to light your path, and it is up to you to decide whether or not you are willing to see the light and trust the journey onward.

CHAPTER 3

⌒

Permission to Rage

Where there is anger, there is always pain underneath.

—ECKHART TOLLE

Anger is an acid that can do more harm to the vessel in which it is stored than to anything on which it is poured.

—MARK TWAIN

Thump. Thump. Thump. Pause. *Thump. Thump. Thump.* A young girl is bouncing a plastic ball in a dusty courtyard. This is her only toy. It is her most treasured possession. The thumping is low and muted against the soft-packed dirt. She wears no shoes, but she has grown accustomed to walking on her calloused feet. She tucks her cropped, raven-black hair behind her ears when the strands fall repeatedly around her cheeks as she plays. Suddenly, a shout from inside the small, thatched-roof house behind her interrupts the thumping. Her mother emerges from the doorway with large metal shears. She screams at the little girl, berating her for making so much noise. In her rage, she cuts up the plastic ball and starts to force the pieces into the little girl's mouth, while the little girl stands dumbfounded, tears streaming down her cheeks.

This girl was my mother. I have heard this story many times, as it has been seared into my mother's memory even after so many years, and each retelling of it seems to validate her experience. It was real. And she survived.

Anger. Rage. Explosion. What would prompt a mother to treat her young child this way? What failed to happen that resulted in this type of traumatic interaction? Stories like this, and the many you have probably heard from family and friends, explain why we, as members of Asian diasporas, may struggle so much with the emotion of anger. Of all the emotions we may try to hold with awareness and intention, anger can feel like the most difficult to manage. It ignites a surge of adrenaline and threatens to destroy everything in its path. This is why we may fear the anger of others so much. This is why we may fear our own anger so much.

When we fear our anger, we work hard to avoid it. We minimize it or brush it off; we convince ourselves that we are too sensitive or moody or irrational. We will do anything to ignore the messages that our anger is trying so desperately to share with us. We build walls around it, seal it off, and drop it deep down within ourselves and pretend it has been dealt with—except our anger doesn't disappear. It hides in spaces that now live outside of our awareness, waiting and wanting to reveal and unleash itself at unexpected times.

My maternal grandmother was born in rural Taiwan, the youngest daughter of seven children. Hers was a farming family, and she was expected to work on the farm until she married. With no more than a third grade education, there were few options available to her aside from marriage or manual labor. My grandmother rarely shares details from her childhood. All we know is that there was likely abuse, trauma, and a great deal of pain. Often these life tragedies dot a whole lifetime of feeling mistreated, scared, and alone, which can cause a great deal of anger even if it is hidden beneath the surface most of the time. In cultures and societies in which anger is villainized, it often has nowhere to go except for deep inside. The intergenerational roots of anger and rage fueled by trauma can run deep for many immigrant families and raise the question, "How do we heal so we can break cycles of intergenerational trauma across generations?"

In this third chapter, I invite you to dive deep with me and give yourself permission to acknowledge your anger and rage. The very thought of this might make some recoil. It might make you scared. It might trigger internal self-talk that this is a dangerous, ridiculous, and terrifying thing to do. But hear me out. I am not recommending for us to *act* with anger and rage at others or displace our anger toward the people around us. Instead, I am suggesting that we give ourselves permission to *experience* anger within ourselves and see it as a red X marking the spot for deeper exploration. There is so much richness and knowledge hidden beneath that anger—knowledge that most of us have never had a chance to uncover because we have been running and hiding from anger for most of our lives. I am encouraging us to honor our anger as wisdom so that we can use it to protect and preserve and as a tool for creating a life that builds empowerment.

⌒ REST STOP ⌒

Does your family have stories of how pain reverberated through generations, perhaps through the expression of anger? How did these expressions of anger impact people, relationships, and dynamics within your family? How would your family have changed had people started developing awareness of their anger and pain and actually worked toward healing it?

THE WORLD VERSUS YOUR ANGER

There are so many forces pushing up against you. Some of them are societal values. Others are cultural values. Regardless, these forces tell us stories about who we should be and how we should behave, as if we were actors in some grand play. I would like to impolitely call BS on this, particularly regarding messages about anger. My entire life as an Asian American woman has consisted of playing out this script time and time again. I ignored my inner knowledge in order to speak the right lines or play the right character, all the while betraying my own deep knowledge that something did not feel right. The following are just a few of the messages you may have received about your anger, and I am sure there are many more. I encourage you to uncover the messages you have internalized about your anger and explore how they impact you.

Be Nice

The world would have us believe that being nice is the most important virtue, because it keeps the peace and makes people comfortable. It smooths over and reduces risk of conflict. Being told to be nice also encourages us to ignore our anger signals even in the face of injustice or mistreatment. In our society, anger has been labeled as "not nice" and so it is considered a "bad" emotion. We were never taught that you can be respectful *and* angry. You can be assertive *and* angry. You can communicate your point *and* be angry. When Asian children are being told by classmates "I can't play with you because you have coronavirus," the nice response might be to ignore it or walk away. But what if the respectful yet assertive response is to call the behavior what it is? Tell them that it is racist and ask them to stop.

As a parent, I am no longer teaching my kids to be "nice." I am instead teaching them to be kind. Perhaps this is semantics, but the idea of being nice triggers a feeling of having to smile through one's teeth while screaming on the inside, disavowing real anger and internal experiences for the comfort of others. I am no longer doing this; neither am I expecting my children to do so. My goal now is to honor my anger in effective ways. I am asking myself, "How can I understand my anger enough to use it for my benefit and move me toward my goals or core values?" That's how we harness the power of our anger.

Be Mentally Strong

Within Asian cultures there is significant stigma against having strong emotions. It is almost as if once you are labeled as "too emotional" or "too reactive" or, even more pejoratively, "crazy," it then gives people justification to disregard your feelings or opinions. Many people have shared with me that whenever they express anger, people start labeling them as "crazy." What a convenient way to gaslight another's emotions. When we are made to believe that our anger is not valid, we start to doubt and question our own anger. We start to believe that our anger is unfounded or not real. We begin to mistrust the very anger that was designed to protect us from the outside world.

There may also be family members who struggle with anger management or mental health difficulties and, as a result, are often feared or written off. Being associated with those "out of control" family members is a way in which people have asked you to shut down or control your anger. *Don't be like your father. He's*

always angry. Stop being like that cousin. They are not stable.
We encounter so many negative messages about anger that we
fear being labeled like those from our community who have been
ostracized because of their emotions. Our culture and society have
done all of us a disservice by writing off anger as an emotion that
cannot be trusted.

Be Silent

As Asian immigrants, most of us have experienced the impact of
stereotyping and racism as a pervasive part of our lives. For Asian
Americans, the model minority myth has created a caricature of
individuals who are hardworking, compliant, highly educated,
and passive in the face of mistreatment. The struggle with this
well-known trope is that it may also impact how we show up with
our anger and how the dominant culture expects us to engage in
the face of mistreatment or injustice. When society views you as
part of a community that will not speak up, rock the boat, or fight
back, this places you in a dangerous position. Not only are you at
higher risk of being stepped on, mistreated, or passed over, but
when you do speak up, the reaction and retaliation can be even
harsher. You are called unprofessional, a sore loser, or not a team
player.

The importance of Asian Americans in the United States has
largely been left out of history books despite the fact that we were
critical to the expansion and growth of this country. Our "invisi-
bilization" has allowed people to benefit from our knowledge,
sweat, and blood with little representation and legal protection.
It was not until 1982 and the murder of Vincent Chin that Asian
Americans became a protected class under federal civil rights
prosecution. If for much of history the society in which you live

has failed to value you, protect you, or keep you safe, expressing your anger becomes a perilous act.

〜〜〜 **R E S T   S T O P** 〜〜〜

What messages have you received about your anger over the years? How have these messages stifled your ability to feel and express your anger? What spaces feel safe enough to express anger, and which spaces are unsafe?

ANGER IS WISDOM

Anger, as an emotion, offers deep wisdom and knowledge if we are willing to uncover that knowledge and capable of doing so. The problem is that anger is an emotion that sits on the surface. It is mercurial, it grabs easy attention, it sparks energy, and it tries to discharge action. If we stay with the anger on the surface, it can serve as a distraction, keeping us stuck in cycles of dysfunction with people and systems. Uncovering the wisdom of anger requires you to sink deeper to darker, more tender and painful spaces, places we often would rather forget and avoid. It is these very painful, vulnerable spaces that our anger is often trying to protect us from because they are so difficult to approach.

We can think of anger as data points for important situations in our lives. Anger is normal and critical for survival. Often it serves a function and has a purpose, even if that purpose is outside of our awareness. Anger is also a seed that has the capacity to evolve and grow into an invasive plant if it is not properly tended. Finally, anger gives strength, motivation, drive, and power, and it can spark courage in the face of adversity. All of this is available to us, but too many of us are too afraid of our anger to harness its important benefits or are unsure of how to do so. Let's explore some important functions of anger.

Anger Is Protection

One of anger's primary functions is to protect us from the outside world. We are constantly interacting with other human beings, who have their own motives, wants, and needs. This does not make them bad or malicious people; they just have different goals and objectives than we do. So, all day our conflicting needs and wants are colliding against each other as we are trying to achieve our own goals. This collision point is where anger becomes critical. Our anger can often become a signpost that someone has crossed a boundary of ours, intentionally or not. And when these boundary crossings occur, they can trigger such reactions as frustration, irritation, or pure anger. Anger serves to protect your boundaries and prompt you to do something about it.

Anger has another function: letting you know when you have been subjected to inequity or unfairness, especially as women, people of color, and other marginalized groups. When we are mistreated or dealt an unfair hand, this can trigger necessary and righteous anger. Civil rights activists have written and spoken about righteous rage providing fuel for the necessary and critical work toward racial and social equality. Writer and activist James Baldwin wrote, "To be a Negro in this country and to be relatively conscious is to be in a rage almost all the time." Anger serves to protect you from mistreatment and injustice and challenges you to take a stand when you need to.

Finally, anger can arise when a goal you have been working toward has been thwarted. We all have been in a situation in which we have wanted something badly. And for some reason, we hit a barrier or obstacle that threatens to take all of that away. Some of us will blame ourselves and feel disappointment or sadness. Perhaps we may give up entirely. But others of us may feel anger—anger that something stands in our way. As a senior in college applying to graduate school, one of my mentors and professors said flatly to my face, "You won't ever get into any PhD programs in psychology. You are a nontraditional student. You should get a master's degree first." Instead of taking his recommendation to heart and criticizing myself for being silly enough to think I could be a competitive candidate, I got pissed. This anger fueled me to email professors from prospective programs, to study their research prior to our interviews so that I could quote their own study results, and to do everything I could to prove my mentor wrong. Anger can protect your goals and dreams and give you the emotional power to make a way in spite of potential obstacles or barriers.

Anger Is Preservation of Self-Worth

When we are mistreated, our mind takes these experiences in two possible directions. We either internalize the mistreatment as validation that we are flawed, unlovable, broken, and incompetent, which leads to feelings of sadness, depression, and hopelessness. Or we question and challenge this mistreatment because we know we deserve better. When we know we deserve better than how we are being treated, we can feel that anger. Without this innate knowledge that we are worthy of more, it is more likely that we blame ourselves rather than experience anger toward the people or systems that mistreat us.

Someone once said that "anger is a reminder of the parts of me that love me." It is the part of us that emerges to protect the ego, self-esteem, or identity. It is also the part that fights against the negative messaging we receive every single day. Anger protects me from people who glared at me and my Asian children at the grocery store during the COVID-19 pandemic. Anger protects us from people who would rather blame us than take responsibility for their decisions. Anger protects us from the messages of advertising agencies telling us that we are never pretty enough, thin enough, cool enough, or valuable enough. Anger is what keeps me from believing the constant messages that I am lesser than and I should know my place or stay down. Anger is the part of myself that knows my worth.

Anger Marks the Spot: Dig Here

If you look up the phrase "anger iceberg" on the internet, you often will find an image of an iceberg with words all over it. At the tip of the iceberg is the word anger, and underneath the water's surface is a large list of other possible emotions that exist beneath the anger. Anger is called a secondary emotion because it often arises in reaction to some other, more vulnerable or tender emotion that our minds are trying to protect us from. Anger might be shielding us from some of our core fears of being inadequate, incompetent, or unlovable. Sometimes it is easier to deal with anger, which is in the business of blaming, projecting, and discharging negative emotions onto other people, rather than face the more painful, vulnerable emotions within ourselves. This is why anger functions like an X on an old treasure map, marking the spot where the riches lie. Anger tells us that there is something important here and it's time to start digging; it is the clue that something is worth investigating.

When my partner and I were first married, something about

him upset me, repeatedly, no matter how hard I tried to contain it. Every time it happened, I would feel burning rage rise to the surface, and I would break out into a cold sweat. This thing that made me so angry? Socks. My partner had this pesky habit of taking off his socks and discarding them throughout the house, often not as a pair. I would find socks nestled between couch cushions, under beds, and in random corners of the house. We would argue repeatedly about these socks, and my partner would promise to try to put them in the hamper, only to repeat the fight a few weeks later. We were locked in this battle for a few years, wondering why his "best efforts" were not working. In hindsight, it feels hilarious now, but back then, it drove me up a wall.

Several years into our marriage, I finally took a step back from my anger and curiously wondered why this simple act would trigger such a seemingly disproportionate response within myself. It was only then that I realized I was interpreting his carelessness with his dirty socks as a deliberate sign of disrespect. My partner's inability to pick up his socks conveyed to me a sense of lackadaisical disregard for how hard I worked to keep the house clean. It also made me feel that I was being taken for granted and unseen in our relationship. If he loved me enough, I thought, he would care enough to pick up after himself. Beneath the anger were feelings of being disregarded, overlooked, alone, and taken for granted. In my own therapy work, I came to understand that his lack of verbal gratitude and acts of carelessness triggered my own memories of my mother feeling taken advantage of and disregarded by my own father. All of these realizations helped me see the true roots of my anger toward my partner. Once I was able to see that, it was much less about the socks and much more about my unmet need for words of affirmation and recognition for my hard work. With this awareness, we were finally able to unlock from our anger and move forward from this battle. An additional bonus is that errant socks no longer trigger me.

⟋⟍ **R E S T   S T O P** ⟋⟍

Can you think of times when your anger helped you? How did you decode that experience of anger into helpful knowledge? What function did the anger serve in those moments? Can you recognize moments when your anger served as a signpost to explore deeper? What emotions revealed themselves beneath your anger?

ANGER PITFALLS

One of the key elements of being able to experience and express anger effectively is having safety within our relationships. If there is safety, then we do not need to fear our anger or the anger of others. We can process it as information rather than a threat. But, if we lack safety in our relationships, then we are more likely to hide that direct anger away and use other strategies to manage our anger.

While these alternative (and sometimes maladaptive) strategies may have helped us cope when we were younger, as we move into adulthood, they can often become pitfalls. These pitfalls, which we will explore below, can sometimes obscure the wisdom of our anger. They keep us from seeing with clarity why we are angry and what needs to change, and prevent us from asking for that change in ways that can be well received. Instead, we become so distracted by the sensation of anger and the mental gymnastics involved in managing it that we may struggle to find the wisdom beneath it. Some of these pitfalls are direct aggression, passive-aggressiveness, relentless pursuit, and rage.

It is important to note that many of the ways we individually react to our anger can often point toward trauma responses from earlier parts of our lives. Trauma responses can be seen as the ways we react to threat or fear. Common trauma responses include fight, flight, freeze, fawn, and feign:

- Fight is direct confrontation. If someone punches you, you punch back.
- Flight is trying to run away from the threat.
- Freezing is the act of feeling immobilized or dissociated, struggling to act at all during the threat.
- Fawning is the response of complying with the attacker to avoid future attack.
- Feigning is making oneself smaller or weaker in order to evade further attack.

While a full discussion of trauma and trauma responses is beyond the scope of this book, it can be helpful to identify your typical trauma responses when you feel under threat, as this can help you understand how you might show up under conflict or in the face of anger.

One way to explore the patterns of your trauma responses is to observe how you react under stress or threat. Do you reduce or increase your activity level in the face of a threat? Do you become more or less engaged? Do you find yourself struggling to make decisions when under stress, or do you tend to become aggressive and combative when stressed and angry? Do you become deferential and people-pleasing when under threat? Do you find yourself complying with others and more willing to give up your wants and needs when others are angry? All of these are helpful questions to explore to understand how you might tend to respond under threat. Sometimes the people closest to us are able to identify which types of trauma responses we tend to gravitate toward under stress, because sometimes they bear the brunt of it! It is also possible for us to react with different trauma responses depending on the people involved, the context, and our level of perceived safety in that situation. The next time you feel overwhelmed, stressed, or panicked, pay attention to how you engage with the people around you. You might discover a lot about yourself in that moment.

Anger and Direct Aggression

In this pitfall, we're locked in a pattern of directly confronting or battling another person when angry. Some people come out swinging, especially when they are angry. Often these individuals see the world as having only winners or losers, and they set out to come out on top every time. The problem is, this form of anger expression ends up causing everyone else around them to shut down, or else it causes escalation, especially if the person on the receiving end is also in fight mode.

Direct aggression is also more concerned with being right and winning the argument at hand than with digging deeper to discover what might have caused the anger in the first place. This anger response style reflects the fight trauma response, as perhaps the person learned early on that if they approach a situation with calm or back down, they might get attacked instead. So, gloves up and ready is their approach.

This form of anger expression is also what society and communities are most fearful of and the reason why we are encouraged to mistrust or ignore our anger. Can you imagine what a world would look like if all of us were direct confronters? We would never get anything done during our waking hours! What we as a global community don't realize is the difference between the emotional *experience* of anger and the emotional *expression* of anger as a behavior. We are capable of experiencing anger without acting on our anger and harming property or people in the process. But some of us, especially those who struggle with anger management, might not have learned the necessary skills to know how to experience anger without discharging it directly into aggressive behavior.

Anger and Passive-Aggressiveness

You are likely familiar with this term, but what is passive-aggressiveness exactly? It's a set of behaviors that indirectly express aggression, anger, or discontent. It can be expressed through non-verbal behaviors, social isolation, deliberate exclusion, behind-the-scenes gossip, and more. This strategy may be employed by those who were not allowed to express anger in the past or who have been retaliated against when they expressed their anger directly. Individuals who have been traditionally socialized not to openly express anger may employ passive-aggressive techniques because it is more subtle and socially accepted than direct anger expression.

This can look like arguing about dishes with your roommate when you are actually upset that they still have not paid their share of the rent, or screening all of your parents' phone calls because they insulted your partner during Lunar New Year dinner. The problem with passive-aggressive behavior is that it does not offer any clarity as to why we are angry or communicate to others about our anger. Instead, passive-aggression drops smaller land mines all around the relationship in the hope that the person we are upset with accidentally steps on them. When the land mine is tripped, it results in another conflict that allows us to discharge the anger that had been bottled away beneath the surface.

Anger and Relentless Pursuit

Have you ever been in an argument in which the other person looks disinterested and is trying to end the conversation, which then causes you to lean in harder and push to resolve the conflict right then and there? It's necessary to mention relentless pursuit as a pitfall because at some point in time either we have been relentless in our expression of anger or we have been on the receiving end of it and could not seem to get out of the argument despite all our best evasive techniques. This pitfall reflects a fight response style in which an angry person persistently tries to fight through the conflict in order to reduce the emotional discomfort of relationship conflict, often driven by insecurity or anxiety about the relationship.

This activated mode can either lead to escalation or cause an imbalance in the relationship, in which the other person starts to shut down and withdraw. When this dynamic occurs, clear communication is less and less effective. The nervous systems of both parties are so overwhelmed that they will struggle to re-regulate each other or within themselves. In this state, we are less likely to effectively understand what our anger is communicating. In fact, we are so distracted by the fighting that we don't have the focus to identify the true problem.

A note on these pitfalls: There is nothing wrong with you and it is not your fault if you engage in some of these pitfalls when angry. We all do. In fact, these are strategies you had to adopt in order to survive. With new awareness of them, you can now question whether they are working for you. Some may be useful in certain circumstances, while others may not. But be gentle with yourself as you are learning new ways of approaching your anger and sharing them with people in your life.

Anger and Rage

When we silence or ignore our anger, we push it away, often outside of our conscious awareness. This is where our anger turns into rage, when the seed of anger burrows and grows roots. Rage is the network of stories and memories that we have created to house the collection of past hurts that we hold on to. Rage is what we tap into when we bring up past transgressions and pain that have nothing to do with our current experience of anger. It is the recycling of anger that happens over and over because there is unresolved anger living there.

The problem with rage is that it can be explosive and unexpected because it often exists outside of our awareness. Anger is experienced in the here and now, a reaction to something occurring in real time. But rage can be triggered by here-and-now experiences and make us react in ways that seem out of proportion to the current situation. Have you ever reacted with intense anger to a situation or person and completely surprised yourself? It is possible in those moments that your anger has tapped into a deeper rage that is demanding your attention.

Uncovering the roots of our rage can take time. They can be based on your personal experiences and have intergenerational links. If you struggle to acknowledge your anger, consider meeting with a mental health professional or even starting a rage journal, which you can keep private. People often think that acknowledging their anger makes them more explosive; in fact, the opposite is true. When we allow ourselves to validate and acknowledge our anger or rage, it might actually provide a sense of relief or release. What is actually more problematic is hiding our rage in places where it becomes difficult for us to access and understand. When we push anger and rage outside of our awareness, we lose the ability to respond to them with intention and learn the important messages hidden within them.

────── REST STOP ──────

Consider for a moment how you tend to respond when you experience anger. Do you feel drawn to respond in a certain way? Does it make you feel explosive, combative, and energized, or does it make you feel scared, withdrawn, and shut down? Did any of these anger pitfalls resonate with you? Why or why not?

LET'S START DIGGING

Most anger management strategies follow a similar format, involving techniques that rely on developing awareness of our anger, calming the nervous system, exploring the meaning of the anger, and creating change with this knowledge. What I offer here is not a huge departure from these strategies, but it does provide an easy template for exploring your anger and uncovering the knowledge within it.

I've been asked in the past, "What does healthy anger expression even look like?" In response, I tell them that experiencing anger (an emotion) is different from anger expression (a behavior). When my kids are experiencing anger and are trying to express it, I have two rules: You cannot hurt other people or yourself, and you cannot damage property. If they break these rules, then I will need to intervene to keep them or others safe. Other than that, they are free to express their anger in the moment how they please. Sometimes my kids will cry, yell, scream, punch pillows, run around outside, or just pout. I find that the same rules apply to adults. These strategies work to process the anger through the body and eventually calm the nervous system.

Once the nervous system has calmed down, the ultimate goal is to decide whether we need to do something in response to the message that our anger has sent us. If so, then a healthy expression of anger translates to assertive communication. It is where we connect the dots between (1) "I feel angry," (2) "I need my body to move through the anger," (3) "What is my anger trying to tell me?" and (4) "I need to share about what caused my anger so that others will understand what I need."

Step 1: Name Your Anger

You cannot tame what you cannot name. Because anger is often an emotion shunned by families, cultures, and society, it is also an emotion that is most likely to be hidden away. Sometimes we are so effective at hiding anger that we might even struggle to recognize it in ourselves. We try to be so "nice," and the thought of being angry at someone is so threatening that we push it outside of our awareness.

I would like you to realize that we are likely to be angry at every single person who touches our lives, even those people whom we love dearly. This is completely okay. You can feel angry that your kids demand so much of your time that you are up late at night scrolling mindlessly on your phone so you can have a moment to yourself. You can feel angry when your coworker repeatedly talks over you even though you consider yourself to be their friend. You can be angry at your partner, whom you love intensely, for always doing the one thing that annoys you, despite frequent reminders. All of these seemingly small situations can create surges of anger within you throughout your day.

What you can start doing today is naming that anger. Some people just say it out loud: "Wow, I am really pissed off at my kid right now because he drew all over the couch with a permanent marker." You can own the anger so that it does not need to own you. You can also name the anger by journaling about it. Allow yourself to write unfiltered thoughts and frustrations in a book that is reserved just for your eyes only. This act of acknowledging your anger helps you accept a natural and valid part of yourself and keeps the anger from being driven underground, where it might fester into rage.

Step 2: Calm the Body

A calm body gives the mind stable ground for exploration and curiosity. Anger can make us feel out of control. It is an emotion that sends surges of powerful hormones throughout the body. Anger can propel us to react quickly and strongly if necessary. But most of the time, we don't want to unleash our anger and hurt the people around us, even those who caused the anger in the first place. In those situations, we need to actively manage our body's anger response in order to keep everyone from verbal or physical harm. This is why calming the body is a necessary step in understanding your anger. Because the body, when activated in fight or flight, will struggle to consider different perspectives or reach deeper for more vulnerable emotions. It will want to stay on the surface replaying the anger and fight or avoid and run away.

Many self-regulation techniques are available. I offer some below and encourage you to test and explore different calming strategies that work for you—even those you may discover outside of these pages. Calming the body is a sensory and physical experience, which is why when we calm the body, we must pay attention to the body and the here and now.

Sensory Grounding: Take a moment and draw in a few deep breaths. Then, start to cue your attention to your different senses. Taste. Touch. Sound. Smell. Sight. Take notice of each sensation in your body. Stay with your body even if your mind or anger tries to lead the focus of your attention away. Just pick a sense and refocus on it. You can even place a small piece of chocolate or a mint on your tongue and focus on taste for the entire exercise.

Progressive Muscle Relaxation: This exercise involves the progressive tightening and releasing of the muscles of your body while engaging in deep breathing. There are many guided exercises online you can use to help you through the exercise. This exercise is great for children, too! If you are at work, excuse yourself and go to a bathroom stall or somewhere private and just breathe and slowly contract or tighten different muscle groups in your body. Follow your breath in and out until your body lets go of the vise-grip hold that it might have on you.

Physical Activity: When our bodies are surging with stress hormones, one of the most efficient ways to process that stress and emotion through the body is to move. After a long day, I understand that moving your body may be the last thing you want to do, but exercise can help you release the buildup of stress hormones that have been coursing through your body all day. Lace up those shoes and go for a brisk walk. Schedule a high-intensity workout class. Go hiking with a friend. There is so much benefit to moving the body that is more than just physical.

Step 3: Dig and Explore

If anger is the X that marks the spot, then we must turn toward our anger, once our bodies have settled, and start digging. Your anger exists for a powerful reason. My therapist likes to say, "Don't waste a crisis," meaning, don't let an opportunity pass you by when you could have learned something in the struggle. Becoming angry is a way for you to learn how to listen and recalibrate your life if necessary. If you do not give yourself a chance to explore what the anger is trying to tell you, you miss out on that powerful knowledge.

If it's hard for you to access more vulnerable emotions, consider the iceberg. Look at each of those words beneath the iceberg and ask yourself, "Do I feel hurt? Slighted? Insulted? Betrayed?" Give yourself permission to sink beneath your anger to some of the more tender emotions. Beneath our anger often lies pain or hurt or fear, and when we can turn toward those emotions, we can perhaps understand what our needs and wants are.

Step 4: Accept or Act

Once you have uncovered the true reason for your anger, you are left with a few choices. You can (1) change nothing and stay in the anger every time the trigger occurs, (2) accept the situation and work to reduce the triggers and/or reframe your perspective to manage your emotional reaction, or (3) act on this knowledge and communicate or plan for change.

As I mentioned in chapter 2, my father and I have a complex relationship. We love each other deeply, but we also can trigger each other intensely. There are times when I must accept that I cannot change my almost-seventy-year-old father and his traditional mindset. In these moments, I choose to set boundaries that reduce exposure to my triggers and know when I need to disengage to calm my nervous system. I also work to reframe or reinterpret his actions, which are rarely malicious but can be expressed in hurtful ways. Reframing our perspective requires us to ask, "How else can I look at this situation so that I might shift how I feel about it?" When we are angry, we are in fight-or-flight mode, which narrows our ability to take multiple perspectives and think in alternative storylines. When I am able to remember that my father's intention is never to harm, it helps me reframe his words in ways that allow me to move through my anger more effectively. Notice how I did not say, "I no longer experience anger." Instead, my goal is to move through my anger, realizing that I will sometimes get angry, it will pass, and that feeling and acknowledging my anger will not destroy me or the people I love.

However, there are other times when you must speak up and communicate your anger. In these cases, anger transforms from being an emotion that is experienced into an action: communication. To answer the question "What do healthy expressions of anger even look like?" a simplified answer is that one goal of healthy anger expression is to prompt assertive communication, because it takes assertive communication to protect a boundary, to communicate harm that you have experienced, to speak up about unjust and unfair systems, and to self-advocate. Anger provides the knowledge and the fuel to courageously and assertively communicate, which serves to protect you and show that you value yourself in a world that may not consistently value you.

MOVING FROM ANGER TO ASSERTIVENESS

In this exercise, we are going to try connecting the dots between the experience of anger all the way through to engaging in assertive behaviors to self-advocate or protect our boundaries. This exercise can be used for all situations in which you might experience the emotion of anger and hopefully help you see with more clarity the important knowledge your anger is trying to impart to you.

1. What was the activating event?
2. What specific statements, behaviors, and actions made you angry?
3. Curiously wonder why these statements, behaviors, and actions made you angry.
4. What emotions are sitting beneath your anger?
5. Would communicating how these statements, behaviors, and actions impacted you help prevent future triggers or anger?
6. If yes, is there safety in this relationship to communicate this impact effectively?
7. If yes, then create an action plan for what you would like to share, the impact that it had, and offer tangible ways in which

the other person could show up differently or the situation could be improved to reduce future conflict.

8. If no, then consider whether there are boundaries that should be put in place to protect you from these triggers or if there are mental reframes that can help you accept the anger-inducing situation and move forward.

Review: Did your action plan work? Was it effective in reducing future boundary violations? Why or why not?

* * *

As we end this chapter, I hope you now understand why anger might be a difficult emotion for you to embrace. I also hope you see why anger is a mighty and powerful emotion that can transform your life if you are willing to unlock its message. So much of our fear surrounding our own anger is steeped in how uncomfortable it can make others feel. But if we are able to calm our bodies before we speak or act, we are truly able to give ourselves more freedom and more choices in how we show up in our anger. We also are much more likely to express our anger in ways that move us closer to the goals and life we want. When we finally give ourselves permission to feel our anger and rage, we remind ourselves that we matter, and that the world cannot deny us of this fact.

CHAPTER 4

Permission to Say No

A candle lights others and consumes itself.

—CHINESE PROVERB

You are not required to set yourself on fire to keep others warm.

—UNKNOWN

I was born on July 26, 1983, in Tai-nan, Taiwan. After my birth, the date and time of my arrival was given to an astrologist or fortune-teller of sorts, who calculated my fate and offered three names to my paternal grandparents to select from. But along with the names came a warning: The timing of my birth was a bad omen for my parents. To this day, I still do not know the details of this warning. I only know my parents were told that if I remained by their side, I could bring them misfortune. Back then, it was not unusual for a family to hear this type of news and send the infant to a relative or another family to avoid the potential calamity. This prompted my paternal grandmother to begin pressuring my mother and father to send me away to be adopted by another family.

My mother was twenty-four years old at the time, existing in a culture that valued her opinions and boundaries far less than those of her husband—or any man, for that matter. In fact, it was a culture that repeatedly tried to set her in her place and reminded her that "no" was not a valid response. Individuals who were more senior in status or age had free rein to impose their will on her life. They had the power to demand that she give up her infant daughter based on the unfounded premonitions of a fortune-teller. It was my mother's forceful "no" that averted what could have been a traumatic, life-altering event. Despite the voices pushing her to comply and to obey, she found strength within her faith and her will to refuse.

While this is an extreme example, it speaks to the external forces and pressures that we constantly face in our lives. When the wants of others press up against our own needs, it forces us to confront the complex boundaries that exist within our relationships. The unfortunate truth is that many of us may not have realized that boundaries exist and, beyond that, are allowed. Interpersonal boundaries can be difficult to see, can change based on the person or context, and can be redrawn to allow for exceptions or changes within a relationship. Boundaries can sometimes feel like a moving target as they are difficult to understand, define, communicate, and enforce; because of this, we may be completely confused about them. Boundaries must be taught and modeled in order for them to be learned and understood.

In this chapter, I extend my fourth invitation on this journey, and potentially one of the most important: permission to say no and to develop boundaries that allow us to preserve ourselves in the midst of our relationships. Many members of Asian diasporas have shared with me that they struggle intensely with boundaries. I believe one of the reasons for this struggle is because we are living between cultural worlds that hold different perspectives on boundaries, so setting boundaries as an act of preserving the self may feel like a betrayal of our cultural upbringing or even those we love.

But what if we could love our people and still have boundaries? What if, without boundaries, we run the risk of souring our relationships with resentment and reactivity when we can no longer take people overstepping our borders? Consider: Having boundaries allows us to love our people well, and to do so, we only need to develop the right muscles.

~ **REST STOP** ~

Turn inward for a moment and ask, "How do I relate to boundaries?" Do you struggle with understanding your boundaries and where they begin and end? Do you have a hard time saying no when you want to? Do you find that you are more often than not allowing your boundaries to be crossed even when it causes you great distress?

Cultural Adjustments

It is important to consider that what we believe to be problematic boundaries may actually be just fine for someone else. In many Asian cultures, it is not uncommon for parents and children to sleep together in the same bed until the children are much older or out of necessity due to space limitations. In Japan, families may bathe together fully naked until middle or high school, and this is viewed as healthy and a form of family bonding. Notice how these practices might be viewed as negative, problematic, or even harmful through a Western cultural lens. As a result, when

I work with clients in assessing the impact of their boundaries, my primary question is "Do you find this boundary or lack of boundary to be a problem?" If my client believes that the boundary is not problematic or distressing, then I honor their perspective and follow their lead.

When clients reveal that certain boundary crossings cause them to become upset or angry or share that they are feeling overwhelmed and stressed out when they fail to protect their boundaries, I begin to help them uncover the problematic boundary and build the necessary skills to approach these boundary crossings differently. I mention this because some clients have shared with me that some mental health professionals, who are unaware of the cultural nuances that impact boundaries, may actually pathologize certain interactions or customs from cultures with which they are not familiar. The words "enmeshment" and "codependency" are sometimes used to describe Asian families in quite pejorative ways. This is not to say that enmeshment and codependency do not exist within Asian families, but that we must be careful in labeling things as harmful if they are not seen that way by clients. This is why it is so important that we evaluate the impact of boundaries through the eyes of the person who is impacted.

BOUNDARIES WITHIN ASIAN CULTURE

The concept of boundaries is heavily influenced by our values, cultural frameworks, and beliefs about how individuals should engage in relationships. The Eastern cultural framework of inter-connectedness will likely result in different boundaries between people than within the Western framework of individualism—of course, the boundaries and borders between people may look and feel different between cultures. This is why so many of my clients express that setting boundaries makes them feel like they have done something wrong, and you may feel the same.

Asian culture exerts unique influences on boundaries that might impact members of Asian diasporas differently from Asians who never left their homelands. Because members of Asian diaspo-ras are immersed in two cultures, we are frequently exposed to the ideas and values that sometimes feel completely opposed to each other. We might simultaneously value independence and intercon-nectedness and as a result feel stuck. In traditional Asian culture, there might be some untrue narratives surrounding boundaries you have heard and felt when you tried to hold your own needs in tension with the wants of others, especially your family and par-ents. We explore some maladaptive narratives about boundaries here in order to develop our boundary negotiation skills within important relationships in our lives.

Boundaries Are Disrespectful and Selfish

In cultures where interconnectedness and self-sacrifice for the com-mon good are prioritized, the idea of creating boundaries might be labeled as selfish. The very act of saying no within the hierarchical framework of some Asian cultures might be seen as an act of dis-obedience, defiance, or disrespect. In some cases, the act of saying no actually invites more pressure and coercion, as boundaries are not viewed as something to be respected; rather they are structures meant to be bulldozed or broken down with persistence and attrition.

This is why, for those of us born to Asian immigrants, setting boundaries might be so difficult—there may be no shared belief that boundaries should even exist, because self-sacrifice for the collective benefit is viewed as the honorable and dutiful path. When your parents have sacrificed so much, the act of saying no can induce an incredible amount of guilt and shame.

⌒— REST STOP —⌒

What were your early experiences with boundaries? Did the adults in your life protect and honor them, or did they ignore and bypass them? This might give you some clues as to how you might approach boundaries in the present.

Boundaries Reject Family and Culture

Asian American clients have shared with me that when they try to set boundaries, especially with their parents, they are accused of being "too American" or "too individualistic," as if the act of setting boundaries is a rejection of our collective culture. Boundary setting may feel as though we are no longer abiding by the expectations of our culture. In truth, when we set boundaries that have not previously existed, suddenly we are reducing or cutting off their previously unrestricted access to us. It may feel like we are choosing ourselves over family, and this may be seen as deeply shameful.

However, we must examine the cost of allowing unrestricted access. We must question how an inability to say "no, I don't want to," and "no more" impacts how we continue to show up in our family relationships. The deeply embedded hierarchical structure of Asian communities can make it feel like we can never say no to an elder, even in the face of abuse, mistreatment, or toxic behavior.

But at what cost? What if, instead, we did the harder work of teaching others where our boundaries are and showing them how to be in relationship with us in a way that works for *both* of us?

——— R E S T   S T O P ———

What is the cost of rejecting our own wants and needs in order to stay connected with others? Is there a boundary in your life that you have avoided? What fears live in that boundary space? What are you worried you might lose?

Boundaries Are Unloving and Uncaring

What if I told you that boundary setting is an act of love for yourself *and* others? Boundaries offer us a way to honor ourselves while loving each other well. Many of us have been told that our boundaries were established out of spite, frustration, or intolerance of others and that setting boundaries is unloving, uncaring, and cold. The need to prove our love and care by dropping all of our boundaries can be a red flag, signaling either that this other person has a poor understanding of the importance of boundaries or that they are adept at manipulating others in order to get what they want—both of which are dangerous and problematic if left unchecked.

I always tell my clients that we would not set boundaries with people who we have no intention of staying connected with. There would be no point in communicating and explaining a boundary with someone you were planning to avoid for the rest of your life. Instead, boundary setting is actually an act of love for yourself and for others that helps us figure out how to love each other well. It may seem counterintuitive that boundary setting is an act of love, but we show love to others by being clear with how to engage us well. As Brené Brown likes to say, "Clear is kind." Boundaries are a gift to your future self because they protect you and give you opportunities to ask for what you need in a relationship and boost the likelihood you will receive it.

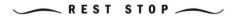

REST STOP

Do you struggle to set boundaries with your loved ones? Does prioritizing your energy, time, and health trigger a sense of guilt? If you looked inward, what is a deep unmet need of yours that you believe is worth protecting?

Boundaries and Burnout

Neglecting your boundaries in order to prove your love is one of the quickest paths to burnout. The idea that we must sacrifice ourselves completely in order to show love and care is causing many of us to burn our candles from both ends. Many people—Asian American or otherwise—are at the brink of physical and emotional burnout because setting boundaries is not part of their vocabulary. As I write this book, millions of people are feeling the weight of burnout as a result of a pandemic. Many of these individuals are in the helping professions or are caregivers who have others depending on them. If given a choice, they will sacrifice themselves for others. They also end up in my office so anxious that they cannot sleep at night. They are so overwhelmed that it affects their performance on the job. They are so exhausted that they sometimes wish that they did not wake up in the morning. Boundaries are what give us the ability to conserve our resources and protect ourselves for the long-term goals we have in this life. Living without boundaries is like thinking that a sprint is a great way to start a marathon. At some point, we run out of fuel and find ourselves wondering why we are so deeply unhappy.

WHAT ARE BOUNDARIES?

We've discussed some of the cultural challenges involved in establishing boundaries, but are we clear on what they really are? Boundaries can be thought of as the space that exists between people. It is the space where one person ends and the other begins. So much happens within that liminal space between two people where your physical body, emotions, thoughts, needs, wants, and responsibilities are separate from the physical body, emotions, thoughts, needs, wants, and responsibilities of the next person. These boundaries are what allow you to be you and me to be me when we are in the presence of each other.

I often have people share with me that they don't want to have to deal with boundaries. They are too messy. Too hard. Too annoying. And I will jokingly reply, "That is achievable...if you become a hermit." If you decide that you have had enough of this complex world and subsequently choose to live by yourself off the grid, you would probably lessen your need to understand and develop boundaries because no one would be interfering or pressing up against your boundaries anymore. However, it's unlikely that being a hermit is part of your life plan, so in order to remain connected and in relationship with others, we will always be impacted by boundaries, whether we enforce them or not. There will always be people who try to reach across the space between us in search of something from us, be it our time, energy, resources, bodies, or ideas.

One way to think about boundaries is to imagine that within you there is a well of resources consisting of your time, energy, attention, and focus. Your boundaries protect that well from thirsty travelers who might come along and try to drain you of all your resources. Instead, you might charge a fee to allow them to have a drink. Or you might set up some barriers to keep them from dipping too freely into your well. These boundaries limit the number of people who have access to your well and keep you feeling replenished and full. When we control and limit who and how many people have access to us and for how long, it frees up energy for us to direct it to the places we actually want to invest in.

However, if you don't realize that your well is valuable and worth something, you might not realize you need to protect it. You might leave it unguarded, allowing an opportunistic person to drain your well to make an extra buck. You might not say no when you are down to your last cup because you might feel guilty for putting yourself first.

Boundaries Provide Safety and Protection

First and foremost, boundaries offer us protection from outside forces. For example, you are sitting in an almost empty subway car late at night and someone boards the subway and decides to sit right next to you. The hairs on the back of your neck stick up as your body reacts to someone being physically too close for comfort. As your mind and body react to this boundary crossing, you might be prompted to physically change seats or to get off at the next stop. These physical boundary rules help govern the day-to-day interactions that we might have with others. When someone engages with us in an unusual way, it prompts us to pay attention and possibly react, if necessary, to keep us safe.

The function of boundaries as safety and protection can also be seen when we are around people who treat us poorly or inappropriately. There are times when perhaps we are around family members who do not understand boundaries or have different rules of engagement. In Asian culture, it is not uncommon for extended family members to comment about your weight or your eating habits or ask intrusively when you are getting married and having children. When this occurs, it can trigger an emotional response in you, alerting you to a possible boundary crossing. This emotional reaction may cause you to disengage from the conversation or decide that you will only attend the family gathering for an hour. These actions help you to reestablish and maintain your emotional boundaries to keep you psychologically protected from the inappropriate questioning of your family members.

When we ignore our protective boundaries, we put ourselves at risk for future violations, because the people around us may have no idea they have crossed the line. They may not realize that a rule of engagement exists and are left clueless about how to engage with you well in the future. Boundaries exist to keep us physically and emotionally safe.

Boundaries Conserve Emotional Energy

When our boundaries are crossed—especially when they are crossed repeatedly—we can get upset, which drains a lot of emotional energy. As we get upset over and over because the same boundaries keep getting crossed, it can be physically taxing as our stress levels begin to build. Sometimes this stress may manifest as physical symptoms, including inexplainable stomach symptoms or pain, back or chest pain, panic attacks, muscle tension, trouble sleeping, changes in libido, headaches, or low energy. If we then fail to recognize, communicate, and maintain our boundaries, we place ourselves at risk for repeated emotional upset, anger, resentment, and rage. Over the long term, this is an exhausting way to live—all your resources will be tied up in managing your emotional upset over these violations.

Although it may be easier to bypass a boundary or ignore times when others cross our boundaries in order to keep peace and avoid potential conflict, boundaries are the gift we give to our future selves. When we are intentional and proactive about setting boundaries, we actually recalibrate the relationship early on. We reestablish the rules of engagement in clear and tangible ways, which can reduce future violations. Each time we allow an important boundary to slide, we hurt our future self and future interactions with that person. By punting the hard conversation to a future time and date, we run the risk of allowing our frustration to brew, making us much more likely to explode when the stakes get higher. Although it can be hard—setting real boundaries takes time, patience, and consistency—your future self will thank you.

⌣⁓ R E S T   S T O P ⁓⌣

Do you feel constantly drained? How might your boundaries explain your levels of exhaustion? Are there boundaries that you may need to enact in order to protect your energy, time, and resources or to increase your sense of safety and protection around certain people?

Boundaries Communicate Self-Worth

We all have finite mental resources that allow us to meet our goals and feel empowered in life. And then there are other people, like those who insist on having free access to your well, who also want to use your finite resources to meet their own goals and objectives. If we continually give our resources up for free, it conveys a message that we are either unaware of the value of our resources or unwilling to protect them. Our unwillingness to protect our boundaries may stem from several reasons: wanting to keep the peace, being a people-pleaser, fearing conflict, or believing that we do not deserve to stand up for ourselves.

Those who really struggle with boundaries also commonly struggle with low self-esteem and self-worth. Often, they have been told that they are not worthy of being treated with respect or valued by others. Sometimes, this is due to experiences of trauma, abuse, or neglect, which can seriously impact identity and perceptions of self-worth. When we feel unworthy, we may be glad that someone—anyone—reaches out to us. We may be willing to do anything for some attention or a feeling of belonging. In order to maintain that connection, we may feel pulled to lower our boundaries and give those people what they want in order to feel wanted and needed in return. In an ideal world, people would see your generosity and protect it. The reality is that when we fail to have boundaries, we are at much higher risk of being taken advantage of.

When we assert our boundaries, we are saying, "Yes, you matter, but I matter too." There is real strength in the act of your refusal to remove yourself from the relationship for the sake of the other person. Holding our boundaries becomes an act of self-love, reinforcing to ourselves that we are worth protecting and our resources are valuable. Boundaries show others that we believe we have value too.

Boundaries Preserve Relationships

Learning the art of boundary setting means practicing the art of effective communication. These two skills go hand in hand. Just knowing your boundaries is not enough; you must at some point communicate your boundaries to others in ways that can be understood. Boundaries have gotten a bad reputation because often we wait to set boundaries until we are pushed to the brink and become reactive; reactive communication is often not effective communication, which is why people come to believe boundary setting can damage a relationship. However, the opposite is true. It may be that we only go through the effort of setting boundaries when the relationship matters enough for us to preserve it.

When we fail to set boundaries, our frustration and anger about the boundary crossing is never communicated clearly to the other person; as a result, we have to hold that negative emotion inside of us each and every time we come in contact with them. These negative emotions and possible future boundary violations might decrease our desire to be around this person in the future. When this person is someone you can't avoid contact with—a parent, a partner, a family member—each unfortunate interaction leads to death by a thousand cuts. This is why setting boundaries acts as a preservative of important relationships. How can we stay in relationships while denying ourselves of our needs? With boundaries, we are able eschew the pent-up resistance or avoidance that can sour a relationship over time.

Are there people you started to avoid because of repeated boundary violations? Who are these people in your life? What boundaries have you failed to communicate and maintain in these relationships? How much longer can you remain silent about these repeated boundary crossings?

TYPES OF BOUNDARIES

Once you can give yourself permission to acknowledge that boundaries are allowed to exist and are vital to your emotional and relational health, you can begin the work of understanding what kind of boundary has been crossed. There are a few basic types of boundaries:

- **Physical boundaries** are the borders of physical space between you and other people. When a physical boundary is violated, it can look like someone who is sitting too close to you in the empty subway.
- **Emotional boundaries** relate to people's feelings and the limits of our impact on people's emotions. When an emotional boundary is violated, it may mean that your emotions are disrespected or that someone has asked you inappropriate questions about your emotional life.
- **Intellectual boundaries** refer to thoughts, ideas, and topics that you might be curious about and how others might respond to your ideas and thoughts. When an intellectual boundary is violated, it may mean that your idea was criticized, ignored, or disregarded.

- **Sexual boundaries** are the limits you have related to the emotional, physical, and intellectual aspects of your sexuality. A violation of sexual boundaries may be in the form of denying ability to consent or in unwelcome comments, touch, or acts.
- **Material boundaries** are related to what material or financial resources you decide to share or keep. Material boundary violations may include excessive borrowing of objects or possessions or using these resources as ways to coerce or manipulate relationships.
- **Time boundaries** are the limits we protect in order to use our time in ways that align with our needs, wants, and values. Time boundary violations can occur when people are disrespectful of our time, demanding time that exceeds what is expected, or asking professionals for their time without compensation.

REST STOP

When you think through the different types of boundaries, are there certain types that you seem to struggle with? Can you recognize when these boundaries have been crossed? How do you know? What do you feel emotionally? How does the boundary violation impact your body?

THE BOUNDARY CONTINUUM

We can think of boundaries as existing on a continuum. Rigid boundaries are inflexible, difficult to break through, and firm. They form a fortress, which is great for protection but quite difficult for human connection. People who have rigid boundaries tend to approach relationships with strict expectations and struggle to adapt to different types of people or situations. For example, someone with a rigid time boundary might become irate when someone is three minutes late to a meeting, such that they cut that person out, deciding they are not worth engaging with. The thinking is, if someone is going to fail you once, they will fail you again. Better build that wall now so you aren't disappointed again—it doesn't matter if there was a good reason for the tardiness. Rigid boundaries do not care about mistakes or accidents. They keep people at arm's length with their boundary walls. Rigid boundaries can be a coping response because we may have been disappointed or hurt too many times in the past. Sometimes the thought of getting let down one more time just hurts too much. So, we keep others at bay, where they cannot hurt us or let us down. We might say it is because we are extremely independent, but it is also because we have come to learn that we cannot trust anyone but ourselves.

On the other end of the spectrum are those whose boundaries are too permeable, diffusive, or nonexistent. In this case, there are no protections or boundaries to shield against the demands, opinions, wants, and needs of others. And as a result, you are often pushed around, disregarded, and stepped on. A permeable or nonexistent time boundary might be reflected by the person at work who agrees to take on every project even if it means that they are overwhelmed all the time and have no time to do their actual job. This person, in their struggle to say no, will implicitly convey to others that they are willing to take on work or projects at their own expense or detriment. They are unable or unwilling to protect their time resources, and as a result, others will take advantage of that, intentionally or not.

So, what is a healthy boundary? It depends on who you are, the situation you are in, your cultural background and values, and with whom you are interacting. This is why boundaries are so hard to learn! But healthy boundaries do have a few important qualities: Healthy boundaries recognize and protect your needs and wants in the midst of all the competing demands in your life. Healthy boundaries are adaptable and flexible.

Adaptable boundaries allow our borders to be redrawn, reevaluated, and reconsidered when different situations or encounters arise in our relationships. **Flexible** boundaries allow those borders to expand and contract fluidly based on the situation. This makes it possible for us to respond with empathy instead of anger when an overwhelmed friend calls us all the time to talk about their struggles caring for an elderly parent. It allows us to offer compassion when our partner is drowning at work and is unable to meet our emotional needs. In these situations, adaptable boundaries help us preserve the relationship but also remind us that our needs do still exist and that, when the time is right, it is important to protect and reinforce them. Adaptable and flexible boundaries allow us to control our boundaries versus allowing them to control us.

It is important to note that having adaptable and flexible boundaries is not the same as having permeable or nonexistent boundaries. Maintaining adaptable boundaries means that the boundaries still exist, you are aware of them, and you are *choosing* to temporarily adjust or shift your focus due to the circumstances that you are in. Adapting your boundaries means that you can still hold people accountable for crossing your boundaries even if you do so at a later time. When talking to the friend who is struggling with elder care, you probably won't stop them during your phone call and tell them they're taking up too much of your time and crossing your time boundary. Perhaps later, during a separate phone call or over email, you can say, "Hey, I realize this is an extremely difficult time for you, and I want to support you as best as I can. But calling me every single day to vent after you finish caring for your mother is getting to be too much for me. Perhaps it is time to find a therapist or support group. Can I help support you in finding these resources?" Flexible boundaries allow our needs to be recognized while helping us adapt to the ever-changing boundary influences on our lives.

REST STOP

Where do you tend to exist on the boundary spectrum, from rigid to permeable? Is there a part of the spectrum that feels safer for you? How might you remind yourself of this spectrum when met with boundary crossings?

HOW TO SET BOUNDARIES

We've arrived at the million-dollar question. How do we effectively set boundaries? Often the thought of setting a boundary triggers enough anxiety and discomfort that we promptly stop there, without trying. We give ourselves an out and decide that our needs and boundaries are not that important. We may tell ourselves, "It's not a big deal. They didn't mean to cross the boundary. Maybe I am too sensitive?" We can apply the skills we learned in chapter 2 here, and work toward tolerating the feeling of discomfort, which the act of setting boundaries can definitely cause. In fact, our ability to tolerate emotional and interpersonal discomfort may actually impact whether we feel confident in setting boundaries with others.

I offer you a systematic method for moving from the emotional frustration of a boundary violation all the way through to reevaluating whether our boundary setting is working for us and recalibrating our boundaries if necessary. Please realize that you may not make it through the steps every time. You might practice the first or second step a few times before moving forward. Give yourself time to think about and practice the different steps until you are ready to go all the way. This is not a competition, and no one is evaluating you. I encourage you to remember that boundary setting is a skill requiring a lot of practice, feedback, and consistency. Do not expect to master these skills quickly or with ease. Instead, offer yourself gentleness and patience as you practice boundary setting first with safe, loving people and then slowly expanding these skills to other people in your life.

When Boundaries Are Not Enough

There may be times when you have communicated the boundary well and maintained and reinforced it beautifully, and the person still does not respect the boundary. In fact, they threaten or challenge that boundary despite your clear communication. If these boundary violations begin to take a toll on your mental health or your perceptions of safety, or they interfere with your ability to live a healthy life, then it might be time to consider whether severing the relationship is necessary, as an act of self-preservation. Often these individuals exert toxic forces in your life. They make you feel miserable each time you interact. You come away doubting yourself and judging your every move. In these instances, after you have tried all that you can to

engage in effective boundary setting, ending the relationship (even if temporarily) may be the best thing you can
do for yourself. A person who is unable to empathize or
understand your boundaries will continue to wreak havoc
on your emotional life for as long as you allow them to do
so. The hard truth is that sometimes saying no isn't enough,
and we need to leave the relationship.

Define the Boundary

It is difficult to set boundaries if you don't know what they are or
if you are unaware of them. It's why we're talking about boundaries now, after we've addressed strong emotions and anger. Your
emotions—in particular your anger—can offer you important
clues that your boundaries may have been crossed. When we first
meet people, we are just learning about their personalities, values,
and interactions with us. This is when we begin forming expectations about the boundaries that might exist between us. Sometimes
the boundary violations are overt, impactful, and overwhelming.
It is so clear that you cannot deny it. More often, boundary violations start small. They begin with small infractions between people, intentional or not.

When I was in training, one of my supervisors started placing
his hand on my back for a second too long. It was enough to raise
an eyebrow, but I was quick to dismiss it. I didn't set the boundary
because I questioned whether it was intentional. I also didn't want
to stir up trouble and appear difficult. But as I continued to ignore
my gut reactions, these boundary violations progressed to suggestive looks and comments about my appearance. My repeated

failure to acknowledge my emotions and anger, as warning signs of boundary crossings, meant that I kept my mouth shut and continued to stomach the discomfort of going to work every day. To this day, I wish I'd understood and known what I know now about boundary setting. I would have saved myself a lot of anger and frustration.

The first step, then, to healthy boundary setting is paying attention to your emotions, not necessarily as absolute facts, but as signals for deeper investigation. Pay attention to how your body responds as possible cues to boundary violations. Does your body become tense, activated, scared, or panicked when you are with this person? Do you become uncomfortable, uneasy, or worried around certain people? Is there a sense of dread when you need to meet them? All of these are cues that are worth exploring deeper when wondering whether these people will recognize or respect your boundaries.

The second step is defining the borders of the boundary. Figure out first what behaviors, actions, or interactions trigger a sense of boundary violation. What is the most permeable or open boundary that might exist within this relationship, and how does it make you feel? Then go to the opposite end and identify the most rigid boundary that might exist between you and this person. When I had my first child, there was a certain auntie (Asian families tend to call anyone who is your elder an auntie) who loved to make comments about my child-rearing practices. When I chose to nurse my daughter for the first few months, she claimed that formula was more filling. When I decided to use cloth diapers with my daughter, she said it was a filthy practice. She basically had a comment for every decision I made. I could hardly stand to be around her. This is when I knew I had to figure this boundary out. My options were:

Permeable (no boundary): Let my auntie keep commenting on
my child-rearing decisions.

Rigid (strict boundary): Cut my auntie out of my life.

The third step is to find the healthy or *workable* boundary for you and your context. In my example, I needed to find a workable boundary because I did not want to cut my auntie out of my life. Remember that we don't usually go through the work of setting boundaries with people we do not care to have an ongoing relationship with. It was my auntie's behavior that was troublesome, but not her entire personhood—this is an important distinction. There were still other positive aspects of her that I appreciated. When we try to find a workable boundary, we are defining how we would need to be treated in order to stay within the relationship. Identifying the workable boundary can be the hardest part, because we must be able to clearly identify what specific changes or behaviors must occur in order for the relationship to continue forward. With my auntie, the workable boundary was to engage her so long as she was able to keep her child-rearing comments to herself.

Communicate the Boundary

Once we have found the workable boundary, we move from the internal work to the external communication of the boundary. This step is often most difficult, because we need to overcome our fears and concerns about how others might react when we communicate a boundary. Often people will say, "I tried. I set the boundary, and they got pissed, so I gave up." Over time, I have developed three principles of boundary communication that I share with my clients (and often have to remind myself of) when they are doing this work:

Expect counterreactions when setting boundaries. Placing a boundary where one did not previously exist might create a counter-reaction. Individuals who are understanding, empathetic, and safe may not have a negative or strong counterreaction. In fact, they might even thank you for the feedback and apologize for the boundary crossing. However, there are others who might be shocked and then angry that you are setting a boundary. They might react in the moment or more passive-aggressively later. When people begin learning how to set boundaries, I encourage them to *expect* counterreactions.

If we set a boundary, we must decide to hold it. This is regardless of what the reaction from the other party might be. I frequently role-play these types of conversations with clients. We practice what exactly they will say and play out different possible reactions. One of the role-play reactions is always a negative, angry counterreaction. Afterward, I ask, "If this strong negative reaction is what you receive, would this boundary still be worth setting? Is this boundary important enough to hold and maintain, even despite the negative reaction?" This line of questioning helps us determine the importance of the boundary and whether we are prepared to enforce and maintain it, despite the pressures to let it go.

Humans prefer predictability over discomfort. We're creatures of habit, and our interpersonal dynamics are often played out over and over again, so much so that it becomes a habit. We prefer this over the establishment and likely discomfort of new but healthier patterns. Sometimes in our effort to set boundaries, we might get locked into conflict cycles that we cannot seem to get out of. When this occurs, I encourage you to literally draw the cycle of conflict that results from boundary setting (see the following example). We need to explore what causes these cycles to repeat again and again. This helps us hypothesize new ways of interacting that might side-step the cycle and set us on the path toward a new way of engaging.

Here's one example of a conflict cycle: Auntie criticizes my decision to nurse my daughter, which leads me to become reactive and angry. I reactively snap back at my auntie, which causes her to become upset and complain that I am ungrateful for her help and how she spends so much time cooking for us before each visit. We begin arguing about how she always makes herself out to be a martyr. The conflict escalates to the point of her leaving. The next time we see each other, it is as if the conflict never happened.

Notice how never once during this conflict cycle was the boundary ever communicated clearly. I never said, "Auntie, it hurts me deeply when you criticize my decision to nurse my daughter. I would appreciate it if you kept these comments to yourself if you decide to visit us." Instead, we took turns reacting to each other but not truly hearing each other or learning how to engage in healthier ways.

These three principles can help to ground us when we communicate boundaries that are not received well. When we communicate our boundaries, it is important to use "I" statements to share impact of the boundary violation, communicate the workable boundary clearly, and offer tangible behaviors that would honor the boundary. For example, I could have said, "Hey, Auntie, I know you do not intend to hurt me, but when you criticize how I take care of my daughter, it hurts my feelings and makes it harder for me to develop confidence in my parenting abilities. I would appreciate it if you no longer made comments about my parenting choices when you come to visit us."

Enforce and Maintain the Boundary

The previous step is not the final step, although it would make sense: We communicate the boundary, they hear it, and we all move on. In some cases, people receive our boundary setting well and agree to shift their behaviors in order to stay in relationship with us. But everyone we interact with isn't going to be understanding and empathetic—if they were, they wouldn't be crossing our boundaries so frequently. When we're clear about our boundaries and they are still crossed, we may become angry and frustrated; our boundary setting apparently didn't work. The greatest lesson here is that setting a boundary also means that when it is crossed, there will be a corresponding consequence that follows. This is the most crucial piece of boundary setting, and one we often forget. A boundary is only as real as the consequence that follows if the boundary is violated.

If you tell your parents to stop asking when you will be married and have children (setting a boundary), but when this line of questioning occurs during your visit, you quietly sit through it, your silence communicates that you are not prepared to hold the boundary and keep others accountable when the boundary is violated. When this line of questioning occurs, you must intentionally remind your parents of the boundary: "This conversation is making me uncomfortable, and I would rather not get upset when I visit you. I want our time together to be positive for both of us. I think it is better that I leave before anyone gets upset." And then you stand up, bid them goodbye, tell them you will visit again next week, and exit. Notice how the enforcement of the boundary did not involve screaming and yelling, but merely reminding them of the boundary and providing a behavioral consequence for the boundary violation (leaving the visit earlier than planned).

Also notice that you didn't threaten to stop visiting if they don't stop their behavior in turn. Setting boundaries rarely goes well when coupled with threats and ultimatums. Boundaries are communicated through words and reinforced and maintained through action.

Boundaries Focus on You

When we enforce a boundary, we should stay focused on *our own* behavior when the boundary violation occurs, not on the behavior of the other person. It's an important distinction and one worth exploring. Focusing on the behavior of others when they violate a previously communicated boundary leads us to become angry, reactive, and triggered, potentially sending us into yet another conflict cycle with that person, which does not reinforce or support the boundary. If we pay attention to our own behavior when the boundary crossing occurs, we now have control over how we will show up and maintain the boundary. Instead of focusing on how that person has yet again upset you, draw the focus of your attention to what you will do now in response to the boundary crossing. This empowers us in the moment to focus on what we have control over (our own actions) versus what we cannot control (the other person's behaviors or thoughts).

Reevaluate the Boundary

I've presented setting boundaries as a process, but it's worthwhile to note that in reality, boundary setting may not feel quite so systematic. It may feel just plain hard. Setting boundaries is a skill that builds on several others, including emotion regulation, effective communication, and identity work. This is why it can feel like setting boundaries is the last thing we want to be doing when we are overwhelmed. However, the irony is that the fewer boundaries we protect, the more overwhelmed we become, which can weaken our ability to set future boundaries. It is a cycle that many of us become trapped in.

In my work with clients, whenever they work up the courage to set boundaries with people in their lives, we always return and talk through it. We dissect what happened. What was said. How did each person react? What was the takeaway message? What worked? What did not work? What surprised you about the conversation? This is precisely how to grow and deepen relationships with others, through updating our mental frameworks for our relationships and revising our expectations, whether positive or negative. It also encourages us to be honest about the boundaries that some people may never understand and reminds us of how we will choose to show up during those times.

BOUNDARIES ARE ALLOWED TO CHANGE

The idea of shifting, redrawing, or adjusting boundaries may seem like a failure to some of you. It's easy to think that if someone does not abide by our boundaries and we need to shift them, then perhaps we just aren't strong enough to hold the boundary. In reality, we all enter into relationships with assumptions and interpretations that are constantly being revised based on real-life experiences. And there might be times when you decide to sever a relationship after repeated boundary violations, which is a necessary but heartbreaking reality. But there might be other times when you hear another person's perspective or that person starts to change. Or you uncover a bias or deep fear within yourself that changes how you feel about a boundary that you previously clung to. The beauty of growth, healing, and our evolution is that we are encouraged to be in a constant state of reevaluation, even with our boundaries.

I'll leave you with a personal anecdote. My mother-in-law and I have struggled intensely with knowing how to love each other for the sake of my partner, her only son. Our conflicts sometimes have become so heated that it was hard to imagine how we could come back from them. Our generational, cultural, and hierarchical differences caused us so much strife. This tension early on in my marriage resulted in weeks, if not months of no contact. This was the only way for me to protect myself for many years. The walls of my boundary were so thick that there was no way for her to reach me. However, over time we started to communicate our pain, we started to cross the generational divides that seemed to tear us apart, and we just kept trying despite how painful it was to set boundaries, learn how to honor them, and find a path through. We are still learning. We are still messing up all the time. But we have grown and have a much deeper appreciation for each other now. As I began to voice my needs and boundaries, I felt less of a need to hide or distance myself from her. And over fourteen years, I have finally begun to revise my boundaries with her, as she has learned how to understand my boundaries and I have learned how to see her needs. It has been one of the most challenging parts of my life, but despite all my skepticism, it has improved. Boundary work can result in boundary revisions, and that is okay.

THE BOUNDARY JOURNEY

Now it's your turn. This exercise aims to help you work through a potential boundary crossing in your life that perhaps you have been ignoring or avoiding. The best part is that you do not need to act today. In fact, most of our boundary work happens before we make contact with the other person. It is the internal work of understanding ourselves that helps us guide others on how to engage and love us well.

In this exercise, I encourage you to consider a relationship you are struggling with. Perhaps choose a relationship you are frequently feeling angry about, or a relationship you do not feel safe within. Select any person in your life who seems to challenge your boundaries knowingly or unknowingly.

1. Ask yourself a few questions: What are the boundary crossings that might exist in this relationship? How do you know? What emotions live there? Where are they showing up in your body? What do you feel when you are in this person's presence? What is this boundary meant to protect?

2. Define the boundary: What are the most rigid and the most permeable boundaries that could exist between you and this person? What is the workable boundary (the boundary border that you can tolerate, live with, and accept)?

3. Communicate the boundary: Think through the three principles. Are you prepared for a possible counterreaction? Would you hold this boundary regardless of their reaction? What patterns and cycles do you seem to get pulled into with this person?

   - Consider the physical setting where this communication will take place.
   - Think through the specific words you might use to communicate the impact of the boundary crossing.

- What is the specific change or request you are asking this person to do to honor your boundary?

4. Enforce and maintain the boundary: How will you reiterate the boundary? What behavior will you engage in when the boundary is crossed?

5. Reevaluate the boundary: What happened? What worked well? What did not work? Is this boundary workable? Is this boundary aligned with your values and sense of worth?

*   *   *

As this chapter comes to a close, take a deep breath. This topic alone is complex enough to fill an entire book. I hope you realize now that boundaries are healthy, natural, and necessary for a sustainable life. A boundary is not a betrayal of your family or culture, but a refusal to betray yourself and your needs in a world that is always pushing against us. I hope you see that you can still love, respect, and honor others while still also loving, respecting, and honoring yourself. Without boundaries, we will struggle to invest our time, energy, and resources into the things we care most about and to live a value-driven life. As we become more aware of our boundaries and begin the discipline of setting them, expect pushback and realize that those who would rather be with a version of you who is free of boundaries may not be ready for a more empowered version of you—and that is entirely their loss. May you find yourself and your worth embedded within the boundaries that you build, and may you feel the freedom that comes with choosing where your borders begin and end.

CHAPTER 5

⌒

Permission to Take Up Space

If you do not seek to take up space, eventually others will fill it for you.

—Tina Hsia-Ming Wang

How does one reprogram a life spent living in the margins? How do we unlearn the story that we do not deserve to be seen? How do we battle constant feedback that urges us to shrink and be essentially invisible in a world that would rather silence us than see us truly for who we are? I am still learning what it means to be an Asian American woman and daughter of immigrants who is able to give herself permission to exist in full form. In many ways, it feels like I am carving myself out of stone, shaping an amorphous nothing into a fully embodied something, something that has shape, weight, and body. I am carving myself into existence.

What does taking up space mean for us as Asian Americans and members of Asian diasporas? As I teach myself to embody words like "boldness" and "courage," I have had to confront how I seemed to have assumed a bowed posture toward the world. How did I internalize the message that taking up space could be perceived as disrespectful or threatening to others? How did I learn that meeting a person's gaze directly seemed to set off a whole host of threat signals in my mind and body? How did these experiences become so seamlessly woven into my psyche that I did not realize, until now, that there were people in this world who knew they *deserved* to exist without hesitation, while I have never felt this deservingness? Have you?

What I can fully name is that I was not born with a reflex to shrink or minimize myself, and neither were you. When my children were toddlers, my husband and I would find them singing, shaking their booties, and dancing around the house or in the grocery store with no sense of self-consciousness. They were still at an age when they remained unaware of the critical eyes of external judgment. Young children can be so blissfully shielded from the impact of others because they are so focused on their own worldview at that tender age. Notice how children in this age group are able to live so expressively and free, fully embodied.

Somewhere along our life journey, we begin to receive messages that we are too loud, too opinionated, too strong, or just too much. We attempted to exert too much influence, and this was not acceptable to the outside world. In response, we make up rules for how we should show up and engage. We limit ourselves out of the fear of rejection or retaliation for taking up too much space. The dominant culture rewards us when our behavior fits their expectations and punishes us when we don't play by their rules.

───── REST STOP ─────

What does the phrase "take up space" stir within you? Do you struggle with living this out in tangible ways? What messages have you received when you have tried to take up space in your world?

As we open this chapter, I offer my fifth invitation: Give yourself permission to take up space and an opportunity to live in full form. Taking up space is an act of physical and psychological embodiment, which is the act of making something visible. Embodiment means taking what is unseen, unspoken, and hidden, and making it visible and acknowledged. I will be the first to say that this idea is scary as hell, especially as a person of color and as a woman. Taking up space means inviting attention. You will be noticed, and you might be attacked in response. As essayist and poet Ocean Vuong poignantly wrote in his book *On Earth We're Briefly Gorgeous*, "Because the sunset, like survival, exists only on the verge of its own disappearing. To be gorgeous, you must first be seen, but to be seen allows you to be hunted." Taking up space forces us to acknowledge that there might be forces that would rather we stay invisible.

For Asian Americans and Asian diasporas, staying invisible became the currency for survival. Asian immigration was seen as such a powerful threat to white "racial purity" and economic opportunity that the Chinese Exclusion Act was enacted in 1882, marking the first time an ethnic group was banned from entering the United States on the basis of race. Our phenotypic traits exposed our "foreignness" and made us easy targets from the start. Most of us have never had the privilege of blending into crowds. During the COVID-19 pandemic, we witnessed a surge of anti-Asian hate crimes and violence, as attackers unloaded a barrage of verbal or physical assaults on many members of our community, Asian elders in particular. It is no wonder that it is hard to take up space with an Asian body. Our bodies have made us targets from the beginning of our existence in the West.

It is imperative that we question whether this survival strategy continues to serve us and future generations. While keeping under the radar allowed our parents and ancestors to survive, does staying hidden help our individual and collective goals, or is there another path? With effort, we can develop the skills to show up differently in our spaces of influence, working through our racial trauma responses to step into our collective power. We can harness our cultural values to empower our communities, instead of encouraging each other to stay silent.

Before we move on, I want to make clear that I am not minimizing the importance of the systemic and structural change that needs to happen so that violent, racist systems are one day eradicated. I believe that we need both large-scale organizational changes to combat racism and injustice as well as individual-level healing and skill development so that we can be empowered to stand in the face of structural inequality. It is the individual growth that I focus on in this chapter and in the work that many of my clients are bravely pursuing.

⟶ REST STOP ⟵

How have your experiences with racism impacted your ability to show up and take up space? Can you remember stories, images, or memories that reinforced a fear of taking up space? How did you make sense of experiences with racism as a child or young adult?

THE FORCES AGAINST YOU

I struggled through writing this entire chapter. Each paragraph required me to wrestle many internal dragons. I often questioned how I could write on a topic that was still such a source of struggle for myself. It was easy to blame a lack of courage as the reason I struggled to write a chapter on taking up space, but as I examined this harsh self-criticism, I realized that it was not a lack of courage

that struck such fear—it was the insidious training I unintentionally received my entire life, training that taught me to remain
small. Any step I took outside of this fear-based framework lit up
all my threat signals. To this day, I am still untangling myself from
the fear and guilt that grip me every time I try to own my space.

So, here we explore some of the programming many of us may
have received over the years. We offer no condemnation or blame
to our parents and caregivers for the ways in which they may have
contributed to this programming; instead, we acknowledge that
they did the best they could with what they had, given their own
awareness and knowledge. For them, the best way to manage the
threats of racism, their othering, and their immigration trauma
may have been to train us to keep our heads down and keep moving forward. We will also explore the societal programming that
has kept Asians in the margins and how that might impact our
ability to dream about what is possible for ourselves and our community. We cannot fight what we do not see. Naming this programming is the first step of unchaining ourselves from its impact.

Cultural Upbringing and Values

When we grow up in cultures that prioritize obedience and conformity, it can be difficult to learn the skill of taking up space.
Instead of being encouraged to speak out, have an opinion, and
challenge authority, we are reinforced for the exact opposite. If you
had a parent who often became angry when you had an opinion
and expressed it, you may have learned that having opinions was
"bad." If you were scolded by your teacher for knowing what you
wanted and communicating it directly, you learned that stating
your needs plainly was something to be avoided. Instead, you were
told to lower your voice, calm your passions, and contain yourself

so that you did not overshadow or overtake others. A culture of obedience and conformity reduces opportunities for us to practice how to take up space and makes us fearful of the risk-taking that is necessary for owning our space. In effect, we learned to reduce, shrink, and minimize ourselves as a form of self-protection and to maintain relationships that we valued.

Within some Asian cultures, we are working against long-held cultural values including patriarchy and misogyny (to name a few) that make taking up space even more difficult. All of these structures assume inherent hierarchies that define what is allowed between people. These patriarchal and misogynistic structures also administer harsh punishments to those who deviate outside of these rules of engagement. A cultural emphasis on conformity is not always good or bad, but when it inhibits one's ability to self-advocate, it becomes problematic. It can take a significant amount of internal work to unlearn some of these cultural frameworks that keep us from taking up space.

⟶ REST STOP ⟵

Were you allowed to take up space as a child? If so, what did taking up space look like in your family? What behaviors and communication occurred when you took up space? How was it received? What cultural or family-based values seemed to support or reduce your ability to take up space?

Limited Possibility and Representation

Representation is crucial for marginalized individuals because it shows us what is possible. My first Asian American psychology professor was a sharp-witted and snarky Cantonese woman who taught graduate-level neuropsychology courses. She was so knowledgeable in her field that she self-diagnosed her own brain aneurysm as it was happening! She somehow had the wherewithal to communicate her diagnosis to her family members before she completely lost all of her cognitive faculties, including her ability to speak. With this information, they were able to rush her to the hospital just in time. Her doctor later reflected that she had saved her own life. My professor's presence, confidence, and formidable knowledge showed me what was possible as an Asian American woman in a field that largely underrepresented my community.

As people of color and immigrants, the act of taking up space may trigger a whole host of threat and fear signals. Sometimes, we are the only Asian or person of color in the room. Not only are we fighting for our own personhood and space, but we may be viewed as representing our entire community in that fight. The lack of representation of Asians in higher-level leadership, politics, sports, media, and elsewhere means that taking up space can be a terrifying and lonely path. Lack of Asian representation in many fields also means that, even if we reach higher levels of influence, we may be gripped with imposter syndrome, which is a feeling of persistent inadequacy even when we are successful. As a result, we can be overwhelmed with fear that we might not meet expectations, we might not measure up, and we might fail to achieve our goals. These fears, though completely understandable, can make us believe that we cannot make mistakes and lead us to strive for perfection, which can derail our performance and growth.

With little to no representation, we might also be forced to continually prove that we deserve a seat at the table. Obtaining a position of influence is not enough; we need to fight to stay there and keep the door open. Unfortunately, if your field is underrepresented by individuals in your community, you may not have the support you need to push through the very real barriers that people of color face. The lack of representation limits our internal frameworks of what is possible for ourselves and can heighten our fears about taking up space because of the cost it might take to get there.

———— **REST STOP** ————

Think about your areas of influence: work, school, friendships, and family. How much representation exists for you, as an Asian? Do you have mentors, leaders, or people who have gone before you who you can look up to? How does having Asian role models or cultural leaders impact what you believe is possible for yourself? How does it impact your thoughts about how much space you can take up?

Model Minority Myth

One of the most formidable forces against our ability to take up space is the model minority myth. Of course, many of us are all too familiar with this stereotype, as we discussed previously. Asian Americans are thought of as compliant, quiet, hardworking, uncomplaining, unwilling to rock the boat, good at school, high-income earners, and a host of other seemingly positive attributes. This stereotype effectively placed Asian Americans on a pedestal to discredit the reality of racism and the impact of racial inequality on Black, Brown, and Indigenous communities, as described by Claire Kim's racial triangulation theory. This theory suggests that Asians are triangulated between Black and white communities in order to maintain racial hierarchies, with white people on top and Black communities on the bottom. Asians are simultaneously held on a pedestal above other minority groups, to maintain anti-Blackness, while being ostracized as foreign at the same time. The model minority myth says to other marginalized peoples, "See, if Asians can make it, why can't you? The injustices can't be that bad. Just work harder." At the same time, Asians are also constantly being vilified as foreign and disease-carrying and told to go back to where they came from, as seen during the COVID-19 pandemic.

Not only does the model minority myth erase the experiences of Asians who are living in poverty and in need of social assistance, it also assumes all Asians are a monolith and effectively pits us against additional racially marginalized groups. While the sociological effects of the model minority myth are beyond the scope of this book, this myth has caused more harm than good, as it has effectively silenced generations of Asian Americans in the midst of their own injustice and mistreatment. It has contributed to our inability to break free from the compliant, hardworking, and passive box we are often slotted into as Asians.

This raises the question: If your community is viewed as quiet and compliant, what happens if you deviate from that expectation? Taking up space as an Asian American looks like fighting against this stereotype each time you open your mouth. It means that the *expectation* of how you show up is different from the *reality* of how you show up, and when this discrepancy occurs, it can be upsetting to those around you who expect your silence and complicity.

Taking up space as an Asian American may mean confronting the reality that there might be retaliation when we own our space. It may mean that others may try to put you back in your place, to remind you to "stay down" because you are supposed to work hard but not be opinionated. You can be a part of the team but not strive to lead it. You are only welcome here if you know your place. The model minority myth has created a narrative that our community likely internalized as a form of self-preservation, and it has also created an expectation of how the outside world may see and engage with us, placing us in a double bind that we must work hard to challenge each time we try to take up space.

—— R E S T   S T O P ——

What is the impact of the model minority myth on your ability to take up space? Have you ever experienced retaliation for taking up more space than expected by others? How did you react, and what did you do in response?

CREATING NEW STORIES

If we have made ourselves small due to lifelong programming and external storylines slotting us in roles we've been encouraged to play, then reversing this programming means learning new stories and challenging ourselves to inspect the existing frameworks and wonder, "What other stories can exist for me?" For many of us, the idea of taking up space may have never been realistic or allowable as a way to build a life that is sustainable and empowering.

Taking Up Space Is Your Right

The opportunity and ability to take up space is a human right. You are allowed to take up space as a way to share yourself with the outside world. You also do not have to ask for permission to exist. You are not a burden or a bother for taking up space. The act of taking up space happens in the mind, body, and voice. When my clients begin to take up more space, changes begin to happen in each of these areas. As we begin to take up more space in our minds, we begin to mentally expand the borders of what is possible for ourselves.

As we begin to expand our minds, our behaviors and actions will follow. I recently shared that I used to struggle with meeting the gaze of strangers. Somehow, I had internalized the message that looking someone directly in the eye was disrespectful. But each time I averted my eyes, I felt lesser than or ashamed, even though the other person was a perfect stranger. So, I engaged in an experiment. Each time I went for a run, I made a deliberate point to look my neighbors in the eye and wave hello. I didn't cross the street to avoid them; instead, I allowed my body to fill some space between us and to make myself visible. The first few times, this was uncomfortable and unnerving. But the act of teaching my brain that taking up space in mind and body was not a threat helped immensely in taking up more space in other areas of my life. Through this seemingly small practice, I was able to rewire my fear signals and learned that taking up space, even in small spaces and small ways, is not nearly as threatening as I thought.

REST STOP

Do you struggle to take up space? Why might this be the case? How does your body respond to authority, power, hierarchy, and whiteness? When do you find yourself deferring or shrinking the most? Be gentle with yourself as you uncover these spaces in your life.

There Is Enough Space—You Are Enough

Our ability to take up space is directly related to our self-esteem and self-concept. When we own our space, we are trusting that there is enough space for all of us, and we courageously believe that we deserve to take up that space. We do not need to be perfect models of self-esteem in order to practice the discipline of taking up space. Waiting to feel better—to feel more confident or be fully actualized—before we begin this practice will only delay our arrival. Instead, the act of taking up space is a dedicated practice of self-worth and self-love. When we take up space, we are saying, "I believe I am important enough to be listened to and to be heard."

In an ideal world, we all would have received messages that we are enough over the course of our entire lives. If we all received these messages growing up, our society would be a much happier, more empathetic, and more supportive place. But, as you may have experienced, many of us were treated to quite the opposite. We were told instead—verbally or through actions (or inaction)—that we were unworthy of attention, affection, and love, and if we wanted these affirming actions, we needed to earn them. So, we spent our entire lives shape-shifting for others so that we could belong and be loved. If you struggle with people-pleasing, which is a posture of constantly being attentive and willing to cater to the wants, needs, and demands of others in order to gain acceptance, likability, or belonging, it may be especially hard for you to take up space because the act of filling a space is anathema to how you usually present—shrinking, minimizing yourself, and acting in ways that benefit the needs and wants of others.

⌣ REST STOP ⌣

Do you believe you deserve to take up space? Do you believe that you have inherent worth regardless of what you do or produce? Are there safe people who encourage you to take up space, ask for your opinion, and listen to your concerns? List these people in your journal or wherever you take notes. We will return to them later in this chapter.

Owning Your Space Does Not Mean Diminishing Others

Taking up space often looks like speaking up for ourselves and advocating for ourselves and those we love. It also makes room for recognition and celebration. Many of my Asian American clients have shared that they struggle deeply with this, and perhaps this is something you have a hard time with, too. Perhaps your instinct is to diminish your own hard work or to engage in forced humility. This makes sense, as some Asian cultures place a strong emphasis on the virtue of humility. You may have witnessed times when people around you were scolded for being boastful or warned about flaunting good fortune or accomplishments. Celebrating or acknowledging your success can also be difficult if you rarely witnessed your parents giving themselves recognition for their own hard work and accomplishments. They may not have wanted to seem boastful, since celebrating individual wins can make others feel diminished. It's important to make a distinction between boasting and recognizing our success. Whereas boasting very obviously minimizes those around us, celebrating success is a validation of growth, overcoming obstacles, and in some cases acknowledgment of the community that helped you achieve your success. We do not take up space to overtake, overshadow, or overpower others. The dominant culture and colonialist structures frame the idea of taking up space in this way—by way of consuming, taking, and reducing the space available for those with less power. They impose a sense of scarcity over what is available to all people—even though there is enough space for everyone. We have been conditioned to be fearful of stepping into our rightful space, because failing to acknowledge our accomplishments and disregarding our worth maintains the power structures for those at the very top. As we work hard to reprogram these narratives, can we consider for a moment that our celebration is an act of protest against systemic forces that want to keep us feeling small? Is it possible that individual accomplishments also reflect communal accomplishment and success? Is it possible that when we take up space by acknowledging success and accomplishments, we may also be empowering and inspiring others in our community to dream bigger and expand their space as well?

————— REST STOP —————

When was the last time you celebrated an accomplishment, your growth, or who you are? How did it feel? Was there hesitation and resistance or freedom and ease? Why might it be difficult for you to be celebrated and recognized? How might staying in the shadows be protecting you? What fear lives in the shadows with you?

THE PRACTICE OF TAKING UP SPACE

We've been thinking through this idea of taking up space; you've given yourself time to ponder the space you allow yourself to inhabit. You're beginning to ask why these rules have been set—those that encourage you to be small—and question where they came from. I encourage you to revisit these mental exercises, this questioning process, each time you feel the urge to hide or shrink. Be patient with yourself as you work through the unlearning process.

Let's begin to move from thought to action and the more difficult task of figuring out *how* to trust in our worth and show up to life in more empowered and visible ways. There isn't a magic formula for learning how to be more comfortable with taking up space. After all of my internal work and helping others through their own journeys, I have come to the conclusion that the real first step in taking up space is choosing to act. However, there are ways we can manage the fear that arises when we consider taking up space, and there are some strategies that can help reduce this fear.

Naming the Fear

As modern humans, we've become accustomed to two types of fear: immediate threats and anticipated threats. In the immediate, we may be somehow physically harmed—a bodily crime or an accident. Anticipated fears are those we predict might happen in the future. Most of the fears we face day to day are anticipated fears.

Anticipated fears keep us from taking up space. We fear what other people will think of us if we speak up in the meeting. We worry we will be unlikable if we self-advocate. All of these mental battles keep us from taking the first step forward and trying something new. One of the first things you can do is begin to identify and name the fear-based storylines that fill your mind each time you consider taking up space. Often these fears are based on emotions more than on data or actual events. When you can see how your fears seem to grip you and keep you from moving forward in your values or goals, it helps you see that perhaps they are not always based in reality. Maybe your threat detection system has been calibrated to be too sensitive. Perhaps you can rewire that system to help you more effectively reach your goals.

Courageously Act

Author and psychologist Susan David once said, "Courage is not the absence of fear; courage is fear walking." This could not be truer as we practice the discipline of learning how to take up more space. There is no way to develop this skill except through intentional and courageous action. Imagine we all have spheres in our lives where we feel more empowered and courageous and other spheres in which we feel more insecure and fearful. When we fear and avoid, we shrink these mental spheres of courage. We send ourselves the message that the feared task, action, or obstacle is too large for us to overcome. Specifically, we tell ourselves that taking up space is too scary and too hard; in effect, we become our own self-fulfilling prophecy. Fear grows and generalizes through avoidance. When we fear something, we instinctively back off and try to protect against the fear. As we back away from the fear, we set up a series of feedback loops that validate our inaction: "See, you couldn't have handled that. Better that you didn't try." However, if we see the fear, acknowledge it, problem-solve it, and pull emotional and social support in around it, we are much more likely to act in the face of fear. The action is what reduces our fear.

There will be times in your life when people will not value you no matter how much space you try to take up. Despite all our efforts to self-advocate, there will be people who decide that we are not worth respecting, valuing, or celebrating. This is where courage comes into play. There will be times when taking up space also means courageously making the decision to walk away and go where you will be valued. This very act is a testament to your value and worth. Television producer, screenwriter, and author Shonda Rhimes once said, "Plenty of people will decide that you can't do something. Plenty of people will decide that this room is not for you to be in. Your only job is for you to decide that every room you are in is a room that you belong in, and to remain there. I always think that's the most important thing—to feel like you belong in every room you're in."

Create Feedback Loops

The powerful by-product of confronting fear with action is that we begin creating feedback loops. By acting, we start to test and retest our anticipated fears. When you speak up during the board meeting, you now get data about how your boss responds or how your coworker reacts. Now, we can work with this data to challenge and question our fears as well as problem-solve new approaches. When we are able to incorporate actual realistic feedback, we are then able to recalibrate some of those fear messages. We are able to say, "Actually, no one said I was stupid when I offered that new idea. In fact, my boss said it had great potential." Courage that produces action helps us tame our fear.

Action also helps us combat fear as it prompts us to learn how to regulate our body's fear signals. In a moment of fear, our sympathetic nervous system is activated. Do we fight or flee? Stress hormones flood our bloodstream. Our nervous system, though, has a counteracting system that can put the brakes on this response: the parasympathetic nervous system. If we engage in deep breathing or mindful noticing of our body in the moment, we can calm our bodies down and re-regulate our physical sensations in the face of fear. When a fearful thought arises and we check it by stepping into our breath, we are telling our body that it is safe, even though we may be mentally terrified. These sensory or physical practices, sometimes called embodied practices, can help us soothe the physical sensations of fear that we might experience when we try to take up space.

Here are a few embodiment practices that you might try when you feel fearful or amped up:

- Practice being aware of your body. What sensations do you experience when fearful or worried about taking up space?

- Focus your attention on your breath. Try diaphragmatic breathing, often simply called belly breathing. Lie on your back and place your hand on your belly; with each inhale, feel your belly rise toward the ceiling, and with each exhale, imagine pulling your belly button toward your spine.
- Wash your hands and intentionally notice the smell of the soap and the temperature of the water.
- Engage in gentle stretching and slowly release tension from the body.
- Lie on your back with your arms and legs extended. Scan your body for tension from your feet to your head.
- Ground your body through your feet. Walk barefoot on a textured surface (e.g., pine needles, grass, round stones, fluffy carpet).

Find Your Hype Team

When I first started my practice in Houston, I was coming out of a season of being a stay-at-home mother, and I was terrified. I was worried about failing and not being able to keep my doors open. I was scared that somehow I didn't know how to be a psychologist anymore. My negative self-talk kept me up at night and made me drag my feet—as we've learned, when we are fearful, we may withdraw, isolate, and hide ourselves. Luckily, I had shared my lofty dream with a few important friends in my life who would not allow my dream to fade. They checked in, asked questions, followed up, and encouraged me to take one small step at a time to start my private practice. One of my friends even offered to sit with me during a meeting to negotiate my rental space.

Facing fear in community might not diminish our fear, but it can create kindling and fuel for our courage. When we realize that we are not alone and that we have safe people who we can be vulnerable with, we might gain a bit more confidence than if we were on our own. I am a huge fan of having a "hype team." My hype team consists of a few close friends who have known me from different stages of my life (childhood, college, graduate school, and beyond). They are brilliant, compassionate, amazing, vulnerable, and real people who receive my fears and doubts with understanding and then remind me of who I am. When the thought of writing a book was too scary and exposing, they reminded me of my purpose for writing. When the first round of constructive feedback from my publisher triggered all my imposter syndrome buttons, they were right there to help me pick myself back up and encourage me to keep going. Facing our fears in community reminds us of what we are capable of and helps us lighten the weight of our fears.

Some of us feel extremely alone. The COVID-19 pandemic especially highlighted the epidemic of loneliness and how it affects us in multiple ways. If this is you, please know that you are not alone. I encourage you to seek out and proactively create spaces to meet like-minded folks, such as virtual writing groups, Zoom-based community circles, or even your local climbing gym or community-based volunteer organization. It will feel awkward at first. It might trigger your fear too. Connecting with others when you feel isolated and alone can be scary, but it is yet another way to take up space and take action. Building a hype team may include interviewing people in your industry who are a few years ahead of you, seeing a therapist for the first time, or taking a chance and asking someone you just met to coffee. You deserve that connection, but you must reach out and make it happen.

TAKING UP SPACE

In this exercise, I encourage you to consider each of the suggestions I offered not as a prescriptive approach to taking up space, but as starting points for your own practice. I encourage you to name your fear, courageously act, pay attention to the feedback loops, and find your hype team. You will hit some speed bumps along the way. But you will arrive at a place of courage and bravery—more so than you ever thought.

Identify the Space

1. What is one area of my life that I wish I could take up more space in?
2. What makes it hard for me to take up space?

Name the Fear

1. What fears are active in this space of my life?
2. What am I most afraid might happen if I take up space?

Courageously Act

1. What small, achievable action can I take to help me take up more space?
2. How did it feel to take one small step?
3. What is the next step I can take?

Create Feedback Loops

1. What kind of feedback am I receiving when I take these small steps?
2. How can I add this data into my action plan?

Find Your Hype Team

1. Who are the people I can rely on to face these fears?
2. What specific things can my hype team support me in as I learn how to take up more space?

*   *   *

As we end this chapter, I will admit that the act of taking up space may never come naturally for me. I have come to accept this. I no longer find fault or blame myself for having to work hard at taking up space. In fact, I see this weakness as a strength, as I am keen to observe when others struggle to take up space and try my best to make space for them to step into. My struggle with taking up space allows me to listen and not jump in prematurely. It helps me remain observant of others. It encourages me to pause without judgment and wait when others struggle to find words and to act. I am now aware of the conditioning that has made my body and mind seize up each time I try to own my space. I am also releasing myself from the expectation of having to take up space all the time, especially when it does not serve me or give me space to take care of myself. I realize now that in order for me to truly take up space, there may be moments when I must choose to prioritize myself and move from fear into action. And though it scares me every time, I try to show up visibly anyway, no matter how small of a step, because the cost of shrinking and minimizing myself is just too high.

CHAPTER 6

Permission to Choose

If you know the enemy and know yourself, you need not fear the result of a hundred battles. If you know yourself, but not the enemy, for every victory gained you will also suffer a defeat. If you know neither the enemy nor yourself, you will succumb in every battle.

—SUN TZU

If you avoid conflict to keep the peace, you start a war inside yourself.

—CHERYL RICHARDSON

Throughout my entire life, I have felt torn between two parts of myself. There was the life I hoped to have for myself and the life I believed my parents visualized for me. These were in constant opposition. The hardest part was that my parents' expectations came with good intentions. Their dreams were rooted in the hope that I would not have to suffer or strive as they did and that my life would be stable and predictable—privileges they lacked when they arrived in the United States. It is difficult to imagine a life where I don't feel the weight of their hopes and the pain of their losses, especially when they came to the United States chasing better opportunities for my sister and me. Knowing that your parents gave up their dreams in order to give you a better chance at living yours has a strange effect on how you think and feel about your own choices.

It is important to say that the freedom to make choices in our lives as immigrants is related to the privileges, resources, and opportunities available to us. Some children of immigrants witnessed the cost of immigration at too early an age and realized that due to the uprooting of our parents' lives, their choices were limited. When my parents immigrated to the US, they lost their entire social support network, which meant they were effectively cut off from financial, emotional, and community support. In an environment with few safety nets in place, their sense of control may have been restricted, and with less control comes less choice. Our parents may have felt that the burden of survival prevented them from true freedom of choice in their lives abroad. Even if your family immigrated with more financial resources and social support, the real barriers of racism, discrimination, and limited opportunities may still have restricted their ability to freely choose their careers and paths in life. Instead, their survival instincts prioritized certain values, such as stability over passion, duty over their own career aspirations, self-sacrifice for the common good over their personal fulfillment—different values than we might hold for ourselves as second- or third-generation immigrants. The clash of these different values can put us at odds with our parents and families when we need to make important choices in our lives.

As children of immigrants, our ability to make choices is shaped by the survival instincts we may have internalized from our parents. If you must survive alone in a new country with no support or assistance, prioritizing financial stability is the only option, even if it means sacrificing personal fulfillment or passion. If you arrive in this country with nothing, your definitions of success and happiness are fundamentally shaped by your experiences with poverty. The idea of exposing oneself to risk and uncertainty would seem foolish to an immigrant who is trying to make sure there is food on the table and shelter over their family's heads. As children of immigrants, we carry these fears and trauma responses sometimes even without realizing their impact. And while many of the cultural and familial values that guide our parents—such as a focus on family well-being, a sense of duty and responsibility toward community, and respecting our elders—may ground us and keep us centered, there may also be values or narratives that are holding us back as we strive to live more authentically and with more freedom of choice.

‿‿‿ R E S T   S T O P ‿‿‿

Have you felt a push and pull between your inner longings and dreams and those that your parents had for you? How did you make choices within that tension? What fears arise when you consider choosing your own path?

In this chapter, I invite you into the sixth portion of our journey: giving yourself permission to choose in the midst of influences from parents, family, community, culture, and society at large. How can we give ourselves permission to choose situations, people, and lives that remain true to who we want to be, and to wrestle through the expectations, hopes, and dreams of others and still find our voice in the noise? The act of choosing is one of the most powerful ways that we can impact and change our lives. Choices are the pathways by which our lives twist, turn, and move forward (or backward) toward things that are either life-giving or depleting. This chapter challenges us to consider how we make choices and what the cost is when we bypass ourselves and choose to live for others.

THE COSTS AND REWARDS OF CHOOSING

I want to acknowledge that claiming our permission to choose comes with a cost. In choosing, you are recognizing that others may not always know what is best for you, and perhaps that you might create conflict if you decide to listen to yourself. It may mean that you need to pursue financial independence in order to be released from the expectation of making choices that please others. Many of the people I work with have shared that it was not until they became financially independent from their parents that they finally had the freedom to make their own decisions— being financially tied to their parents meant that they still owed their parents something, and the debt could always be cashed in against their life choices. This sort of transactional relationship is not unusual in Asian families, as there is a strong emphasis on service, duty, debt, and repayment of gifts and offerings.

In choosing, you may also end up losing support from people you love. Perhaps this means choosing to come out regarding your gender identity or sexual orientation, so that you can live without shame or hiding, and subsequently your birth family is unable (or unwilling) to support you in this regard. It may look like potentially being disowned by your family in order to marry someone outside of your race or ethnicity, or deciding to pursue a career in activism or advocacy work instead of joining the family business. Of course, you will feel the grief and loss associated with choosing to live a life that is authentic and aligned but that your loved ones cannot accept. All of these costs must be acknowledged when we choose to live for ourselves versus others. I highlight these struggles and losses not to discourage you from choosing in alignment with who you are, but to illuminate how large the forces against us are. The pressures keeping us from choosing authentically are not imagined, but in fact, they are strong enough to tempt us to surrender and let others take the lead in our lives.

When we give ourselves permission to choose for our own lives, we gain access to some very real rewards. In consciously choosing, we engage in purposeful values-based living. We are defining what matters to us and living in alignment with those values. We are able to push past external judgments and discern the choices that truly matter to us. In this discernment, we also begin to shape our identity and sense of self-worth, because it is now based on internal character and values rather than the judgment or evaluation of others. The power of choice is that we gain ownership over our lives, and this helps us sustain our choice when the road gets rough. The act of choosing can fortify our sense of determination, grit, and perseverance when challenges inevitably come our way. We are also potentially rewarded with less regret over the course of our lives; we knew that when the decision mattered most, we chose based on the people we knew ourselves to be and the people we hoped to become.

When we make choices for our lives, we are practicing the skills of inward listening and outward discernment. We are learning how to understand our own needs and wants while also filtering the judgment and feedback of others and discerning their importance in our decision-making. This skill must be practiced. It will not come naturally. The act of holding what is true and valuable to you in tension with what everyone else thinks or believes can be a daunting task. Many of my clients wonder how they can stop caring what others think when they have been conditioned to care their entire lives. In this chapter, we will explore and unlearn this conditioning.

⌒ **R E S T   S T O P** ⌒

Have there been times in your life when you chose what others wanted for you over what you wanted for yourself? What were the consequences of choosing what others wanted? What did it cost you and what did you gain by choosing what they wanted? What would you do differently in your life right now if you were to give yourself permission to choose for yourself?

OBSTACLES TO AUTHENTIC CHOOSING

When we make choices for our lives, there will always be external forces that try to shape and influence us. This is a natural aspect of living in community with others. Often, these pressures don't come from a place of harm; in fact, they might be quite well-intentioned. Our nearest and dearest may seek only to offer guidance or advice about our decisions. What they may not be aware of is how their worldviews greatly shape how they make choices. These worldviews are built on their unique life experiences, values, and goals, and fundamentally shape how they show up in their world. In holding so rigidly to their own worldview, they likely possess blind spots for different perspectives that others might value too. And while these frameworks may work fine for them, they may not align with *your* life experiences, values, and goals, and can sometimes lead us astray.

It is these frameworks and mental barriers that sometimes prevent us from authentic choosing. When we make a choice, we are actively selecting, editing, and shifting our lives (hopefully) in alignment with who we are and who we want to become. However, many of us have learned to ignore signs from our mind and body that tell us this choice is no longer working or, in fact, has never worked. It is remarkable how effectively many of my clients silence those signals. They are so used to ignoring their inner knowledge; when they are unhappy or frustrated, they shush their inner voice and label it "weak, too sensitive," or, even worse, "crazy." As we discussed in chapter 4, we have been taught to push through negative life circumstances without complaint. We push ourselves to endure through frustrations and discontent to the point of emotional or physical collapse or burnout. In effect, we create a war within ourselves without even realizing it.

In order to move forward, we have to understand our inner combatant. Here, I offer a few obstacles that get in the way of authentic choosing for first- and second-generation Asian immigrants. I recognize there are many more obstacles that impact us than those listed here—these examples are meant to encourage you to consider for yourself the specific obstacles that may impact you when making important choices in your life.

Guilt and Indebtedness

We can understand guilt as feelings of shame or regret that one might experience as a result of a perceived or actual wrongdoing or violation of moral or social standards. Many of the Asian American clients I see in practice experience guilt, primarily as an overwhelming emotion that gets triggered when they try to make life-altering choices. Whether it is an internalized guilt or guilt induced by others, they often share stories expressing the ways these feelings prompt them to make choices they otherwise would not. One source of guilt for children of immigrants might be tied to our parents' struggle to make life work in a new country. These feelings of sorrow or pain regarding our parents' suffering may incite strong feelings of guilt if we make choices that go against the wishes of our parents, who likely gave up a lot to ensure that we had a "better life."

Alternatively, if our lives are "too good" and we live with too much comfort or ease, we may also experience feelings of guilt because our parents did not get to enjoy these privileges. In the context of our parents' suffering, we may believe that "the least we can do" is to comply with or honor their wishes. We may experience guilt when we choose interests or careers that our parents do not support or that may not provide the financial security we need in order to support them in turn in their old age. We may experience guilt when we choose partners who are from different backgrounds than what our parents expected and preferred. We may feel guilt when we decide to move far away from our aging parents. There are a myriad of touch points over the course of our lives that may prompt feelings of guilt for choosing our own path over following what others expect of us.

———— **R E S T   S T O P** ————

Do you find that your discomfort with the emotion of guilt drives your decision-making? Have you ever tried to please others because it was easier than holding the feelings of disappointment or guilt that get triggered when you choose for yourself? Pause for a moment and let yourself name that guilt. Acknowledge its presence in your life.

Filial Piety

Some cultures, Asian and others, maintain moral values that guide how children and parents should interact. There are different terms in different languages that express how children should engage their parents. In Mandarin this is called xiào or 孝. In Korean the term "hyo do" or 효도 describes a similar idea. In Vietnamese it is known as có hiếu. In English, this term is known as filial piety, which describes a "dutiful respect" that a child is expected to hold for their parents. Many Asian American clients have strong and complicated relationships with the word "duty" when used in relation to their parents. Some carry this responsibility proudly and lovingly, as an overflow of their sense of affection and gratitude to their parents. For others, it can prompt a sense of resentment or obligation that they must hold in tandem with their own needs and wants.

It is also a complex value for members of Asian diasporas, as we are raised in a Western social context in which our non-Asian peers may not feel the same sense of duty or responsibility toward their parents. At times, it has been unfathomable to my non-Asian friends that I might feel guilt for not following the expectations of my parents. The rules of engagement between parent and child can vary widely across cultures. I have certainly had clients share that their immigrant parents would pull the filial piety "card" in order to pressure or coerce them into complying with their demands. Of course, not all parents operate under this mentality, but it does highlight the unique ways in which immigrant parents may engage their children who are raised in Western culture, and the potential conflicts that might arise due to these differing perspectives.

⌒ REST STOP ⌒

Does your culture prioritize filial piety? Does your culture have a term for filial piety? How does your sense of filial piety shape your decision-making? What drives you to uphold filial piety as a value in your life? Is it driven by your close and intimate relationship with your parents? Or is it driven by your feelings of obligation and obedience to role expectations within your family? Give yourself a moment to explore how you relate to filial piety as a value system.

Choosing with Rigidity

There is something clean and simple about making a choice and holding on to it until the end. It is easy for the human mind to accept this type of decision-making—it's clear-cut. You make a choice and never waver. However, when we make choices and give ourselves little to no room for self-reflection, questioning, or revising, we can lock ourselves into a life that no longer serves us. I hear all too regularly arguments suggesting that "it is too late" or "I have invested so much" for reasons why people are unwilling to let go of things that no longer align with the overall vision of their lives. And yet, they are often fraught with such distress and turmoil over their unhappiness or discontent.

Perhaps I can challenge you to consider the cost of choosing with rigidity. I work to help my clients understand that one small shift or change in our lives multiplied over years or decades creates a completely different trajectory. Perhaps you aren't ready to make a big leap and quit your job. That is okay and, in some cases, even wise. But what does it look like for you to introduce practices and activities that bring you creativity and joy during your leisure time? Without giving ourselves permission to choose as an act of growth, and to do so repeatedly, we become locked into behavior and thought patterns that may feel safe and comfortable but leave us feeling trapped. Perhaps this space to explore might help you identify a direction or interest that is appealing enough for you to change course and choose something new.

Giving ourselves permission to choose with *agility* over rigidity means that we recognize that our needs and desires change.

In order to shift out of the old we must overcome inertia and the fear of pursuing the new. Many of us also may have never had this behavior modeled for us. Instead, parents, caretakers, and other community members believed you just endured life, even if it made you miserable: You stay in marriages that bring no joy. You remain in jobs that deplete mind and body. You stay in something even if you don't want to. Choosing with agility is a privilege. Can you give yourself permission to access that privilege?

<hr>

⟶ REST STOP ⟵

Do you struggle with allowing yourself to change your mind? Do you believe that once a choice is made you must endure it at all costs? Do you make decisions from a posture of agility or rigidity? Why do you think you operate from that posture? Where did that perspective come from?

Lack of Authentic Knowing

The final and perhaps most important obstacle to authentic choosing is the lack of authentic self-knowing. In my work as a psychologist, I often say, "I wish I had the answer. I wish I could choose for you. But I can't." My clients usually laugh and acknowledge that as much as they would like me to, I cannot make choices for them. Their biggest struggle isn't that they aren't willing to work hard toward their goals or to make difficult decisions to fundamentally change their lives; it is that they do not know who they are or want to be. In effect, they feel lost when asked what they actually want.

I remember feeling lost in college. In undergrad, I was accepted into a prestigious five-year master's in accounting program and was going to devote the next three years to accounting. But I was so miserable. My parents repeatedly asked me, "What would you want to do instead?" I honestly had no idea, because I had spent my entire life listening to the guidance and direction of others. I had never considered what I wanted for myself. I had never explored my life with openness to possibilities, and in fact my life felt like it had a singular focus, which was to finish school and find a job that could pay my bills. That was it. There was never any consideration of what makes me happy, what brings me excitement, or what I could envision doing for the rest of my life. It wasn't until I took my first psychology class that I found the answer.

As children, if we were encouraged to make decisions and listen to ourselves, we may have had a chance to exercise those introspective muscles that help us make choices that are right for us. We learned how to evaluate and recalibrate our life choices in response to that internal voice. This practice allowed us to develop those self-awareness muscles and gave us confidence in our ability to make decisions. However, if we were often told what to do, what choices to make, and that choosing for ourselves was selfish, we may struggle to know ourselves and trust our inner voice. We might feel uncertain and unwilling to commit to decisions out of fear of making the wrong choice and not knowing how to recover from our mistakes. We instead look to others constantly for reassurance that we are making the right choice.

─── **R E S T   S T O P** ───

When was the last time you knew that you wanted something different for your life? What did it feel like? What was stirring within you? Was it excitement, drive, motivation, passion, interest, or thrill? Did you trust these emotions, or did you feel pulled to ignore them?

WORKING THROUGH DISCOMFORT
AND GUILT

Guilt may not be the only emotion that gets stirred up when we are faced with difficult choices, but for us children of immigrants, it can be a prominent one. We may also feel discomfort or shame when we know that what we really want is in opposition to what those closest to us believe is right for us—or else we risk losing their support. In order to become confident in the act of making choices for ourselves instead of for others, we must learn how to create space and honor these negative emotions. It is imperative that we face these emotions—avoiding them leads us into cycles of self-silencing and emotional upheaval, as we repeatedly try to evade the difficult choices that we know, deep down, have to happen. We lose our ability to listen to our deepest desires, wants, and needs. If we are able to hold the tension of emotional discomfort while also actively making decisions that align with our values, we are at least able to move forward toward our goals. If we can acknowledge the difficulty of making choices but make them anyway, we can move away from the frustration, indecision, and fear that keep us stuck.

I was overwhelmed with guilt when I decided to quit the accounting track to pursue psychology. My parents paid for my college education, and here I was about to make a jump that might flush their substantial sacrifices down the toilet. I knew few practicing psychologists and even fewer who had full and successful careers in this field—none of whom were Asian. It was a gamble, and it felt like gambling with my parents' hard-earned money. But I also knew that if I did not choose psychology, I would have left business and accounting eventually. It was only a matter of time.

I had to question: How would pushing myself to suffer through a career I hated honor my parents' hard work and financial support? If I was honest with myself, I knew that it wouldn't. Since childhood, I had internalized the idea that I needed to secure a well-paying job to take care of my parents in old age. The thought of pursuing psychology triggered so much guilt because I believed that I might not be able to make enough money to support them when they needed me to. It felt selfish and ungrateful to choose my own happiness in a career over my ability to financially support my parents. So, I pushed forward in my business degree, thinking that if I just ignored the deep sense of dread and discontentment, it might go away. When I finally could no longer silence myself, I had a recurring thought: *I will not be able to sustain a lifelong career in something I hate. So how will that help me support my parents in the long term?* I knew it wouldn't. With this realization, I was able to sit with the discomfort of taking all the necessary steps to change my career trajectory, because I realized that the path I was on could not guarantee financial stability either.

Many of the individuals I work with come to therapy seeking help in moving through the natural inertia that comes before great change. The following sections provide a framework for pushing past discomfort and guilt.

Holding Space

Guilt is just another emotion, like anxiety, fear, or sadness. It is a response to any situation in which we believe we may have caused harm or failed to meet a perceived or expected social standard. Like fear, we often have to remind ourselves that we are capable of sitting with, holding space for, and tolerating guilt. It is our very ability to hold the emotion of guilt with intentional space that allows us to critically evaluate what it is trying to alert us to. When we experience guilt, we feel ashamed for something we believe we have done wrong. But the first question we might ask is, "Have I truly committed wrongdoing in this situation?"

Guilt is generally prompted in the event of the following:

1. Our behavior, thoughts, or feelings do not match an external expectation, rule, or social norm we believe others have placed on us.
2. Our behavior, thoughts, or feelings do not match an internalized expectation, rule, or social norm that we have placed on ourselves.
3. Our behaviors have caused actual specific and identifiable harm to another person, whether intentional or accidental.

It is important to distinguish between perceived wrongdoing versus real and identifiable harm toward another. When we have committed actual wrongdoing toward another, the guilt is natural and helpful as it reminds us to reconsider the action, change the action—if we can—to reduce future harm, and move toward apologizing to and reconciling with the person we hurt. This allows us to remain connected to people in our lives, which has been vital for our survival over time. In this situation, the emotion of guilt is effective in maintaining our relationships, making us more aware and sensitive to others' needs, and helps us stay connected with others.

Is Your Guilt Workable?

An alternative way to think about our guilt is to consider whether it is a workable emotion or response. Workability challenges us to question whether or not the emotion helps us move toward or away from the life that we want or the values that we hold. In the case of managing guilt, we might ask, "Does this emotion of guilt help me move toward or away from the values that I hold or the life that I want?" This is especially important when we experience guilt but have not committed actual harm to another, when the guilt comes from a place of feeling as though we have failed to live up to the expectations that others hold of us.

I wrestled hard with my decision to leave accounting, because it prompted me to experience so much intense guilt. Each time I experienced a bout of guilt, I would ask myself whether I would really damage my parents with this potential decision and whether the guilt was drawing me closer to or pushing me further away from my goals. Ultimately, I realized that the guilt I felt was not necessarily an indicator that my decision was wrong or harmful to my parents; rather, it was an emotion that was keeping me from pursuing the life that I wanted.

There are other times when the guilt may come from outside of yourself. Perhaps you share details about a lavish trip you're planning with a cousin, who then questions your choices—they could never do that, they might say, when their parents would benefit from that extra money. In light of this, you may feel deep guilt, although that might not have been your cousin's intent. As we learned above, what you feel is in response to an external expectation or rule, and this should make plain how powerful guilt can be, such that it can rob you of enjoyment and peace. In this case, is the guilt workable, or is it pulling you away from your values and goals?

Let's look at it from another angle. You're planning this trip, but your parents seek financial assistance from you. You decline to help your parents and continue with your trip planning, only to feel guilty after booking the vacation. In this moment, give your-self space to question what this guilt is trying to tell you. If you have a toxic relationship with your parents, you may decide that you are unwilling to support them due to the harmful relationship. And while you experience feelings of guilt, this would not change your behaviors or decision to take the trip. The guilt is not work-able. But if you have a positive relationship with your parents, per-haps the guilt is highlighting to you that your behaviors (taking a vacation while your parents live in poverty) are not aligned with the person you want to be (an adult child who wants to support their parents through financial hardship). The guilt is telling you that there is dissonance between your values and your behavior, pushing you to reconsider your choices. We could call this guilt workable; it's an emotional response that you can use to help you move closer to your overall values or goals with regard to your relationship with your parents.

Notice how understanding the value and function of an emo-tion like guilt requires us to place it within the context of our val-ues, goals, and vision of who we are. For this reason, when we avoid the emotion of guilt altogether or avoid making choices that might conflict with what others want, we miss out on opportuni-ties to understand ourselves better and make choices that could bring more fulfillment or authenticity to our lives.

RIDING THE WAVE OF GUILT

I once asked, "How do you manage the discomfort of making choices that others do not agree with?" Someone responded, "I ride the wave of guilt." I love this visual because it allows us to validate guilt as an emotion that can rise within us, and it can also fall and diminish. It suggests that experiencing guilt may not always be a sign that our decision or choice is wrong; instead, it's a natural response to a relationship dynamic.

This exercise is meant to help you move through any feelings of guilt you might have that do not align with your values or goals. You may want to revisit chapter 1 and your core values to help guide you in this exercise. I encourage you to think about a recent life decision or a decision you made in the past and work through these prompts. See what surfaces for you.

Think about a time when you experienced guilt due to a decision or choice that you wanted to make. Write it in your journal or another document, along with your responses to the following questions:

1. Acknowledge, name, and give space to the guilt. Instead of resisting it, invite it in. Be gentle and tender with it. Be curious.

2. Question what is driving your feeling of guilt. Who do you feel guilt toward? Is it a specific person, or is it focused on a certain rule, framework, or idea? Did you commit actual identifiable harm toward another?

3. If you have not committed identifiable harm, ask yourself if this emotion of guilt is moving you closer to or further away from your core values or goals in your life. Is the guilt coming from a workable or unworkable place?

4. If the guilt is moving you further away from your core values and goals, can you allow yourself to acknowledge it and allow the emotion of guilt to move through you and pass through? Can you make room for other (more balanced, less critical) thoughts?

5. What emotions or bodily sensations rise up in you as you ride through the emotion of guilt? What are some grounding thoughts that remind you of the importance of your decision?

6. Once the wave of guilt has passed, consider how you feel about the decision or situation now. Does the weight of the guilt feel as heavy? What images, ideas, or expectations have you released yourself from?

When we have committed no wrongdoing, we can become fixated on the emotion of guilt and add fuel to it by criticizing or judging ourselves, which leads to a "shame spiral," as some of my clients like to call it. When we can create space between the emotional trigger of guilt and our response to the guilt, we give ourselves more freedom to decide whether the guilt is a workable emotion (aligned with core values or goals) or not. Our alignment with internal core values remains the internal compass in deciding whether behaviors, thoughts, or emotions are effective or ineffective in helping us navigate guilt.

MENTAL CHECKPOINTS

As I learn how to choose with self-knowledge and intention, I have discovered some important frameworks that guide the permission I give myself to choose. I call them my mental checkpoints of choosing; I try to run difficult decisions through each of these checkpoints. They keep me grounded when there is pressure to keep the peace instead of listening to myself. They remind me of the parts of myself that I will not compromise even if it risks disconnection from those who do not understand my choice. I encourage you to see which of these checkpoints resonate with you and perhaps find your own unique checkpoints to help guide your permission to choose. My mental checkpoints are inner knowing, long-range perspective, sustainability, and chosen family.

Choosing with Inner Knowing

When we are aware of what others want, it can sometimes feel easier to default to their perspective, wants, and needs. This is especially true for individuals who might describe themselves as having people-pleasing tendencies. As a recovering people-pleaser myself, it's critical for me to check in with and create space for myself in the midst of my relationship with others.

We often disregard or ignore our bodies when checking in with ourselves; something those I've worked with have often expressed is that they are so used to living in their distracting thoughts that they are rarely attuned to their bodies. We can improve our relationship with our bodies when we give ourselves time to pause and be silent and still; often, our bodies begin to reveal powerful knowledge about how we are responding to situations or people in our lives. Sometimes the body communicates through lack of sleep, body tension, stomach or back pain, or other bodily complaints with no identifiable medical cause. Listening to how your body reacts to situations, people, and decision points is one form of inner knowing I would encourage you to cultivate. This is such a simple practice, but few of us actually make time and space for it. Consider scheduling five minutes at the beginning or end of your day to focus your attention on your body and scan, observe, and be curious about what it is revealing within yourself. Practices such as progressive muscle relaxation, sensory grounding, yoga, and gentle stretching are also wonderful ways to increase your ability to listen to your body. Listening to your body provides knowledge that may not yet have words or language to express, but your body's reactions can inform your choices through a more primal, instinctual source of knowledge.

I was not kidding when I said emotions are a critical part of this work. Being aware of how you feel about certain situations, people, or opportunities can help inform your choices. Some might argue against making emotional decisions. I would generally agree with this suggestion. It is rarely helpful to make decisions when you are in the midst of an emotional tidal wave, as our ability to think with clarity and perspective becomes impacted during intense emotionality. But, once you have ridden the emotional wave and it has passed, do you return to that emotional information and investigate it? Or do you ignore that emotion, labeling it as irrational or unhelpful, and bypass what you felt? It is a combination of our emotional wisdom and rational thinking that helps us make decisions most effectively.

Passing through the mental checkpoint of inner knowing requires the most discipline—you must prioritize and make space for it. It is also the checkpoint that we may most often overlook, because it requires us to step away from the busyness and distraction of our lives. It also means you must face the negative emotions that might live in that space, feelings of frustration, discontent, and isolation as well as sadness and regret. When you allow yourself to sink into that space of knowing, you also give yourself a chance to see with more clarity what is amiss, which helps you start making decisions that can change your life for the better.

⸺ REST STOP ⸺

Do you feel that you know yourself well? Are you able to create space to listen to yourself? When has listening to yourself helped you in the past? What signs and messages did you listen for, and what was most impactful during those times? Can you allow yourself to trust your inner knowing and the information that it shares with you? If not, what do you need to get there?

Choosing with Long-Range Perspective

By the time many of my clients connect with me to begin therapy, their sense of inner knowing has already alerted them that something is not right, something is missing or feels misaligned. They are deeply unhappy, perhaps realizing that they have only one life, and that time is limited. Through the course of my work with them, as they start to make empowering changes and shift mindsets that hold them back, they regretfully share that they wish they had started taking these steps earlier in life. Few emotions are harder to live with than the feeling of regret, especially when we begin approaching the second half of our lives. None of us are capable of predicting when our lives will come to a close, but many of us live as though we are guaranteed many years to come. The illusion of always having a tomorrow can keep us in situations that are not right for us and thus delay our having to make hard decisions. If you knew that your life would end in a year, or two years, or five years, how would you change the way you spend your time?

This mental checkpoint centers on the notion that our current choices have possible impacts over time. Will making this choice matter in a year, three years, or ten years? Will distress over this difficult decision still be with me in that time frame? Placing our life within a longer-range perspective helps us see a fuller picture and understand the scope of impact that this decision has on our lives. A simple visual exercise to try when seeking to regain perspective is to imagine that you are taking a bird's-eye view of life starting with today. Then zoom out to the week and the month. Finally, envision this day in the context of a year or several years. This can help you understand what is worth your attention in the here and now and help you sift through the situations that may be short-term attention grabbers but insignificant in the long term.

My decision to change careers from accounting to psychology fundamentally changed the course of my life. My inner knowing made it quite clear that accounting was not the path for me, although it came easily academically. Physically, I experienced sleepless nights, exhaustion, and boredom because I had no spark or passion for my studies. I needed to translate this knowledge into tangible action, or I'd risk getting stuck. When I finally made the decision to drop out of the coveted master's accounting program, I was overcome with a sense of relief, thrill, and exhilaration— quickly followed by fear, doubt, and panic. Had I just turned down one of my best options for financial stability? Had I disappointed my parents by stepping off the more logical, secure path? It was scary. It was a risk. When I took a step back and looked at all the hours and years of my life that I would spend working as an accountant, I knew that I could not go down that path without seeing what else life had to offer.

Choosing with perspective means understanding your emotional tolerance for the choices that you make or fail to make. I encourage you to ask yourself, "What am I willing to tolerate in terms of the emotions and conflicts within me if I decide to move forward with something that I know is not right for me?" If I had chosen to stick with accounting as planned, my parents would have been pleased. I would have had potential job security. I would have achieved the goal that my parents had hoped for by paying for my college tuition. But I would have started a war within myself. And I believe that it would have caused an emotional breakdown in the future, so massive that it would have taken many months or years to recover. So, the final question I encourage you to consider is, "What is the cost of not changing?" As someone once said, "What you are not changing, you are choosing."

────── **R E S T   S T O P** ──────

Is there an area of your life where you are struggling to engage with intention? Perhaps a small inner voice has been saying, "This doesn't feel right. This can't be it. There must be something more. Something more real, authentic, and right for me." Allow yourself to pause in that space of wondering and questioning. Now, can you imagine staying in this place for the next year, two years, five years, or ten years of your life? Why or why not?

Choosing with Sustainability

Modern life is data. We are inundated with data, information, and knowledge; we're offered all sorts of things to buy, do, and learn to make ourselves better and our lives happier. Except we are less happy now than we have ever been in the past. We have rising rates of anxiety and depression, especially among teens and young adults.

I believe we are struggling with a sustainability problem. It's a theme that comes up among many of the people I work with. My clients share that they feel like they are in the grind and have been hustling their entire lives. They know how to overproduce with a smile, and they struggle to make decisions that allow them to live the lives that they actually want. Making choices sometimes means that we need to choose what to cut out and let go of from our lives. We need to be deliberate about how we choose to live our lives, because running on autopilot or following the herd is making us miserable. Instead of pushing ourselves through dehumanizing jobs or situations, thinking that we just have to survive until the next vacation, we need to realize that how we are living is not sustainable in the long term.

Choosing with sustainability in mind depends on your level of privilege. Our parents may have experienced different levels of privilege that restricted what they could choose to do or not to do. They may have had to work hard for survival. But some first-, second-, and third-generation immigrants have been gifted with being able to do more than survive. When I consider my decisions and choices, I have had to forcibly remind myself to keep the mental checkpoint of sustainability in mind. I have chosen to turn down opportunities simply because I did not want to do them or did not have energy for them, despite the financial benefit they could provide me. I have decided to prioritize my emotional and psychological well-being, even though everything inside of me says that I can just push through. It has been a hard rewiring of everything in my mind that says, "But more is better, right?" Sometimes more means more stress and less peace and not necessarily better quality of life. I have had to critically evaluate the purpose of pushing through. Is it driven by a higher goal or purpose, or is it driven by my fears of not being good enough or of what others might think if I stepped back? We all exist on a spectrum of privilege in terms of what we can and cannot turn down in order to create more well-being in our lives. But if you have the ability to choose to live with sustainability in mind, it may help bring more discernment to your decisions. If you lack the privilege to prioritize your mental health in the midst of your work or home life, are there people you could ask for support and to offer pockets of space for you to breathe and rest along your journey?

Sustainability also means considering whether we are able to stay committed and motivated when challenges arise from our choices. When I choose to do something that I don't really want to do but agree to it due to pressure from others, I always struggle more when obstacles or challenges arise. I become resentful, angry, and frustrated that I need to handle additional unforeseen issues over a decision that I was pressured into making. I struggle to find the grit and perseverance to push through these challenges because I lack ownership over this choice. I also may blame others for putting me through these hardships despite the fact that I agreed to them. Choosing with sustainability in mind reminds us that we will be the ones that must live out our choices day in and day out, not others.

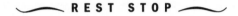

REST STOP

Will you keep sustainability in mind when you consider important decisions? What does sustainability mean to you? What does it look like in your life? What is keeping you from living from a sustainable mindset?

Choosing with Chosen Family

When we make choices, the possibility that those around will not support us is real. This is a reality that many of us must face when we give ourselves permission to choose. We may feel real grief and loss when we realize that perhaps our birth family is unable to accept who we are or our friends seem to fall away when we decide to choose for ourselves. I encourage you to grieve, cry, and mourn these losses, because they can feel like a loss of the most important parts of yourself, like disconnection or rejection from the people you most trusted and relied on. Give yourself that time, and recognize that the mourning process may be ongoing. I further encourage you to look out into your life and consider building your chosen family, which will consist of people who receive you as you are and are capable of sitting within your pain and vulnerability and loving you through it. They might be friends, teachers, mentors, role models, therapists, or others who the universe brings into your life as reminders that you are never alone and that you are already more than enough.

This mental checkpoint is important. I frequently encourage myself and others to connect and ask for support from this chosen family, especially when making difficult decisions. This chosen family will include people who can say, "I know you are scared, but I see potential in you. I believe you are capable of this even when you do not believe in it yourself." This chosen family will remind you of who you have been and what is possible for you. They will offer their support and encouragement when you trip and fall, and they will help you back up again. They will not expect you to change, shape-shift, or perform for them; they will want you to be authentic and real. They will accept and celebrate who you are and learn greatly from you as well. This chosen family will sustain you when you think you cannot go any further.

Choosing with the support of a chosen family acknowledges that there are people who could not show up for you. Perhaps you are estranged from your father, but you have a high school mentor who cares deeply about you. Perhaps you are not on speaking terms with your mother, but your aunt has always been your cheerleader. Look to those who have stepped in during important moments of your life to help uplift you. They might be part of your chosen family. And finally, consider building community around yourself. There are so many nonprofit, volunteer, service, religious, activity-based, and other communities in which you might find some kindred folks. Creating a chosen family helps ground us and cushion the bumps and bruises that we may experience in claiming our freedom to choose.

⟶ R E S T   S T O P ⟵

Do you have a chosen family? Who might be included in this family? If not, are there people in your life who have stood by you, supported you, and encouraged you along your journey? How might you deepen that relationship and connect with them?

*   *   *

As we close this chapter, I hope you have had a chance to reflect on the obstacles that keep you from living the life of your choice. Perhaps you can now see with more clarity the ways in which you struggle to make choices that acknowledge your existence and needs. In the midst of these struggles, I hope that you are able to relate to your guilt with more awareness and consider when it is helping you or when it is actually keeping you from your goals. Take time to create your own mental checkpoints grounded in your values and the life that you are building, so that you can choose with intention and alignment. With practice, I have slowly learned how to listen to myself with more compassion and understanding. Empowered with this inner knowledge, I have yet to lose myself, because I am capable of returning to my chosen path (again and again) even when the outside noise threatens to lead me astray.

CHAPTER 7

Permission to Fail

The glory is not in never falling, but in rising every time you fall.
—CHINESE PROVERB

You may encounter many defeats, but you must not be defeated.
In fact, it may be necessary to encounter the defeats, so you can
know who you are, what you can rise from, how you can still
come out of it.

—MAYA ANGELOU

When I was in third grade, my teacher, Mrs. Burke, called my parents to arrange a parent-teacher conference. Since my parents did not have a local support network or strong community, my sister and I went along and sat in the corner while Mrs. Burke talked to my parents. This was probably the first misstep. My teacher proceeded to tell my parents that I was not doing well in school. In particular, I seemed to struggle with writing and language arts. Like many immigrant parents of that generation, my parents trusted that the school system would provide everything we needed to succeed and left my sister and me to fend for ourselves academically. I was silently tasked with figuring out how to navigate my education on my own, but at the age of eight, I had no idea I was struggling in school. At the end of the conference,

Mrs. Burke suggested that I repeat the third grade. I remember my face flushing and my stomach cramping as if in a vise. A feeling of embarrassment and shame washed over me; it made me nauseous. Already at such a young age, I was confronted with my first experience of failure, and it shook the foundations of my identity and confidence. I felt this failure meant I was somehow broken.

This memory still brings up a lot of pain. It seems to activate a button that causes me to doubt and question my intellect and abilities. It engulfs me with shame despite the fact that my parents ignored her warnings that I would struggle in school moving forward and I never repeated third grade. It fills me with self-doubt and fear every time a new opportunity arises. It made me conclude that because I struggled in school, I must have been the "stupid kind of Asian." This harsh critical voice rears its ugly head every time I try new things or set bigger goals, and to be honest, it's exhausting.

At the time, I had no idea how our immigration journey and being Asian American in a predominantly white school shaped how teachers might have viewed me. I also had no clue that I had internalized the model minority stereotypes that put me into prescribed boxes of what I could or could not be. And even as Mrs. Burke observed my struggles, she never once offered additional resources, tutoring, or tangible support before suggesting that I repeat a grade. All I knew as a child was that Mrs. Burke thought I needed to be held back, and that felt like the most shameful thing for an Asian American like me. This experience altered how I viewed myself and in many ways made me feel like an imposter, even during times of notable achievement or success as an adult. More than thirty years later, I am still working hard to overcome my terror of failure.

Fear of failure is deeply rooted in shame. At some point in

your life, a certain situation or mistake started to shape a story about yourself that those around you either reinforced or failed to challenge. Had my parents stepped in after that meeting and said to me, "I don't believe a word that Mrs. Burke said. You are smart. She just doesn't see it. Let's work together to figure out why you are struggling in school," I believe my interpretation of this event would have been quite different. Instead, there was silence on the drive home. There was silence the next day and every day after for the rest of the year. The failure of my parents to address this incident seemed to suggest their agreement with Mrs. Burke's assessment, that I was not smart after all. I hold no blame for how they handled this situation. In truth, they were probably so overwhelmed and exhausted that they felt powerless as well. But the shame sank deep and started to grow roots in my identity.

As we open this chapter, we embark on the seventh leg of our journey: the permission to fail. And oh my, is this journey a struggle for many of us. This fear of failure exists for all of us as humans, but for Asian diasporas it inhabits unique meaning, pressures, and forces. The notion of failure has altered what we believe we can become and, in some cases, held us back from opportunities to realize our full potential. It has cost us all so much to see failure as something to be feared instead of something to move through and learn from.

Failure triggers a whole host of fears: Fears of inadequacy. Fears of abandonment. Fears of not deserving more. Fears of being unworthy. Fears of disappointing others more than ourselves. In order to shift this framework, we need to proactively reprogram how we understand failure, how it relates to our self-worth, and how it keeps us in a state of inaction.

What would it look like if we embraced failure instead of running from it? How would our lives change if we saw failure as a signpost for growth, evolution, and development instead of as a spotlight of our weaknesses and deficits? How can we, as a people, break from the model minority stereotypes that make us terrified to trip up, make mistakes, or take risks, and instead accept that failure is a crucial step toward things that we believe are worth living for?

———— **R E S T   S T O P** ————

Are there key moments in your life when you remember experiencing shame around failure? What happened? Who was involved? How did you interpret the situation? How did it change how you viewed yourself?

THE MYTHS OF FAILURE

Although it's natural for us to try to avoid anything that creates discomfort, recall our earlier discussion in chapter 2: Our tolerance for discomfort is the key to moving through life with purpose and intention. Remember, by avoiding discomfort, we shortchange ourselves and all that we could be. This is especially important because failure doles out discomfort by the bucketful. The way failure is framed is what makes it especially uncomfortable. Imagine, instead, throwing a party every time someone failed. If we saw it as a milestone and cause for celebration, how differently would we relate to failure as a concept? In reality, our cultural experience of failure becomes wrapped in shame and poisons our ability to access the knowledge that failure can offer us. Shame tells us many lies when we come face-to-face with failure. It says, "If I fail, then I am deeply flawed, messed up, incapable, unworthy, and just plain stupid." It is these messages that make us fear failure so much that we stamp out our dreams, give up on things that feel hard, and make excuses to never start.

Even as I write, I type each word holding my fears of failure in tandem. What if this book fails? What if no one buys it, much less reads it? What if the publisher regrets offering me this opportunity? What if I let everyone down? What if I let myself down? Who will I be after the dust settles? How will others see me? Will they still value me and love me? Fears of failure are rooted in core beliefs about being unlovable, incompetent, and easily abandoned. This is why we struggle with failure so much.

——— REST STOP ———

What makes it hard for you to witness, hold space for, and embrace your failure? What images, memories, or statements are conjured up when you think about failure? Was it a parent, teacher, coach, mentor, or sibling who made you feel shame and unworthiness? How does your body react to this shame? Where does the shame live in your body now?

I recently asked my social media community how they related to the concept of failure, specifically as members of Asian diasporas. They offered a few myths about failure that resonated with me and many others, which we'll explore below. These myths speak to the barriers that keep us from approaching our failure and offering ourselves the space to breathe and move through it. They are cultural and societal programming that trap us into lives that are neither fulfilling nor purposeful. They encourage us to ignore our stirrings, dreams, and aspirations because the thought of having to tolerate the shame that might follow failure is just too much. Before we can move forward, we must look at what's holding us back.

Failure Is Not an Option

Most of my life's successes have been driven by an avoidance of failure. It's a motivational force—so much so that in order to get to a place of action, I would shame myself into anxiety and panic first. It is ironic how something that brings so much distress can also be functional and useful, to a point. But this fear-based mentality also created a deep sense of "not good enough" that burrowed its way into my brain. It transformed every accolade into a deep fear that I would not be able to sustain my success beyond this point. Living in fear of failure means maintaining your place or falling off the pedestal in shame. Any accomplishments only serve to reinforce that perfection and success are the only options. Existing in this way is exhausting. Our cultural upbringing makes this doubly so. For immigrants and children of immigrants, failure is hard to stomach. In many cases, it simply is not an option. The stakes of failure hit differently in our parents' generation, and we felt it too. For some, failure meant unstable housing, an inability to feed one's family, and disconnection from faraway loved ones for months or years at a time. The burden of fearing failure crept up in the scarcity mentality, in choosing stability and safety over passion or interest, and avoiding risks. Some of us hold the legacy of fear inherited from our parents deeply in our psyches and bodies. When you have seen what our parents have witnessed, failure is taken off the table, because failure means that you do not survive.

I make a bold claim when I ask, what if our generation puts failure back on the table? We can acknowledge that giving ourselves permission to fail is a privilege that our parents might have never had, and by keeping the possibility of failure on the table, we acknowledge that it is necessary for growth. What if, instead of fearing failure, we looked for it as a sign that we were challenging ourselves and open to learning? What if failure became a part of ourselves that we could vulnerably share, so that our community did not trap each other in picture-perfect lives of comparison?

───── R E S T   S T O P ─────

Is failure on the table for you? Do you allow yourself the space to fail? Why or why not? What stories have you learned that keep you from allowing failure to be a natural part of your life?

Failure Means I Am Flawed

Fear of failure is rooted in our identity stories, which are bound together by shame. When we experience failure, or feel as though we have, we internalize the experience. We start to try to sort out what about ourselves was the reason for the failure. A lesson I can impart here is that even when we try our best and fight our hardest, the outcome may still not come out in our favor. Understand that experiencing failure or feeling frustrated that the outcome of an action doesn't match your expectations does not mean you are flawed. Failing at something does not mean you yourself are a failure. If we take the emotion out of it, failure is a signpost, which we can use to mark growth and the possibility of learning new skills. Failures are directional arrows pointing toward new and unexpected opportunities. Failures guide our next attempt and next try. The experience of failure hones *how* we try again, but we can't do this unless we are willing to let go of our failed and flawed stories.

───── R E S T   S T O P ─────

Has there ever been a time when you failed and it eroded your courage? Tell yourself the story again. What about the

outcome could you have controlled, and what was outside of
your control? Do you regret not trying again or sticking with it?
What do you wish you would have done in the face of failure?

A Failure for My People

A unique facet of Asian American identity is the model minority myth. We discussed this in chapter 5, and it's necessary to revisit it here. This myth homogenizes the stories of Asian immigrants and eliminates our unique drives, abilities, passions, and cultures. As Asian Americans, we carry the weight of the model minority myth whether we fulfill it or not. We carry the myth by constantly feeling the need to measure up and prove ourselves. We feel its weight when we do not reflect the stereotype and experience isolation or shame as a result. Either way, the Model Minority Myth has inflicted significant and measurable harm on the psychological lives of Asian Americans, which we are still trying to understand.

Many of my clients struggle with themes of perfectionism and the endless chasing of achievement reinforced by the model minority stereotype. Others have been shamed by teachers, mentors, or even their own parents when they did not fit the myth. As a child, I can recall receiving the message that I could prove myself and my right to be in certain spaces by being better and smarter than my white counterparts, something like a "if you can't join them, beat them" mentality. Perhaps you received the same advice, given with the intention of motivating you to pursue excellence so that you would not be looked down upon in the ways your parents might have been. In some ways, it was a way for us to combat racism—if we could simply be better, the dominant culture couldn't find fault with us. So, what happens if we make mistakes, take detours, or fail? Does that mean we have failed ourselves, our parents, and our people? As Asian Americans, we may struggle to hold the collective shame we might feel when we fail, as it might reflect a failure for our families and communities as well.

━━ R E S T   S T O P ━━

Have you ever worried that your failures in school, in the workplace, or within your communities might reflect poorly not only on yourself but on your family, community, or other Asian Americans? What has the weight of the model minority myth looked like for you? How have you had to adapt in order to carry the weight of this stereotype? What have you had to give up in order to carry it?

THE ROADBLOCKS OF FAILURE

Since we are using the metaphor of a journey or quest, I've decided to focus this section on roadblocks, because there are several barriers that keep us from moving through failure effectively. Failure will touch us all in some shape or form, and it is a necessary setback that can be useful—to a point. When it outlives its usefulness, it becomes a hindrance, particularly when it gets wrapped around shame and self-doubt. Let's take some time to deconstruct these roadblocks. Each roadblock below reflects the ways shame turns failures into obstacles. These were developed by observing stuck points—either in myself or in my clients—that keep us from learning the valuable information contained in our failures and letting them go.

Your roadblocks might take on different shapes or forms, so I encourage you to consider the language you might use to describe the barriers that keep you from embracing your failures. Be curious with the mental or emotional blockages that cause you to divert your path as you try so hard to skip over feelings of failure. Avoidance of these feelings will be tempting, but I challenge you to consider what these roadblocks are keeping you from.

The Perfection Roadblock

We all love a 4.0 grade point average, a complete winning record for the season, or a flawless performance review at the end of the fiscal year. Perfection makes us feel in control and safe. It gives us the illusion that our effort is directly related to the outcomes of our lives. After all, how often have we heard "Work hard and life will work out just as it should." But what happens if you work hard and you fail the test, you don't get the job, or you get fired? This shatters our illusions of control and can make us feel untethered and lost. Failure tends to ruin our idealized wishes for perfection.

Perfection is tricky. It can be a barrier to embracing failure, because perfection is only interested in the outcome or end result. It does not honor or care about inner growth or resilience or development of the process. Instead of appreciating the slow, step-by-step journey toward our goals, perfection says we should or must do it in this specific way. It narrows the options for how we can reach our goals and triggers the critical voice within all of us that says, "Why didn't you do this faster, better, or more efficiently?" Perhaps that voice originated from external forces—parents, teachers, other family. They all seemed to say, "It doesn't matter how you get there. You just better end up there." And when we neglect the process and focus only on an outcome, we begin to tie our worth and value to the outcome instead of the growth process.

Perfectionism can also be a false motivator. Many of my clients have shared that even after a "flawless performance," the high is only temporary—then it is back on the treadmill again of self-doubt, fear, and anxiety about not maintaining their performance. The high of achievement fades quickly, and so the cost of maintaining our worth can be extremely exhausting and triggering. For some, these cycles may manifest alongside panic attacks, sleepless nights, harsh inner voices, depression, or a whole host of other mental health difficulties, as you "punish" yourself into perfection. As long as we hold on to perfection as a value, we will struggle to give ourselves permission to fail, because perfection becomes one of the only ways in which we find value in ourselves.

Exploring perfectionism within Asian diasporic communities is a whole book in itself; until that book is written, I encourage you to explore the cost of maintaining perfection in your life and what you may be unable to access if you choose to live with it as one of your core values.

───── **REST STOP** ─────

Do you find that your desire to appear perfect keeps you from taking risks or pursuing goals that you want? What does your perfectionism protect you from? How does it keep you safe and give you a sense of worth or belonging? What do you fear might happen if you showed up less than perfect?

The "Not Good Enough" Roadblock

While perfectionism is focused on only having worth when we are perfect, the idea that we're not enough is rooted in doubt in our self-worth overall. This type of roadblock becomes the constant soundtrack for many people's lives. The personal narrative becomes "I am weak, stupid, unreliable, incompetent." We tell ourselves we are incapable, or unwilling or unable to work hard enough. Where did these interior voices come from? We weren't born with these ideas about ourselves; they were acquired. Take a moment to ask yourself now: Where did you learn them from?

In the same way my encounter with Mrs. Burke planted a seed of doubt about my academic abilities, somewhere along the way, someone planted seeds of doubt within you about your intellect, appearance, abilities, character, and so forth. Failure adds fertilizer to these seeds. It fuels their growth by confirming—even without evidence—that they were right. We truly are all of the negative things people said or thought we were. We can't help it; humans are wired for pattern recognition, and if our minds are constantly looking for evidence to confirm our unworthiness, we will internalize negative feedback and brush aside positive feedback. Instead of seeing feedback as a gift, we will see it as a sign of our unworthiness. Instead of interpreting a rejection as a redirection, we may give up because the rejection means that we are flawed or incapable. Notice how this particular roadblock makes failure a part of our identity by altering what we believe is possible and shifting our behaviors in ways that reinforce how we are not good enough.

Many children of immigrants painfully joke about how they were punished if they received anything less than an A grade on a test or school assignment. They laugh about how their parents had no tolerance for failure. They find commonality in the verbal abuse, shame, or punishment they may have received whenever they were less than perfect. Although we find humor in it, unprocessed anger from these lifelong encounters drives that anger inward, toward the self. This may manifest as self-sabotaging behaviors, making excuses not to try, or labeling ourselves as incompetent because, if we are so, then we can't disappoint anyone. In reaction to our parents' harshness, we may set the bar low so as to avoid being judged. As a client once shared, "It doesn't hurt as much if they don't expect much from you in the first place."

Do you engage in self-sabotage behaviors because you have fears of not being good enough? What are you avoiding because of your "not good enough" roadblocks? Have you set the bar low to avoid the pain and judgment that could come from failure?

The "I Don't Deserve It" Roadblock

There are those who believe they do not deserve success or happiness, either because their self-concept, often demeaned, devalued, and torn down by important figures in their lives, has become eroded, or else they have committed some type of wrongdoing that they are determined (consciously or unconsciously) to punish themselves for. Some truly believe that they deserve to fail, and as a result, they might unknowingly make choices that cause them to suffer or stumble. Often, this is not a conscious choice; even so, people stuck in this mindset find themselves unhappy over and over again and do not know why. I call this a roadblock because it is separate and distinct from perfectionism and the feeling of not being good enough.

If you struggle with this roadblock, you may feel like you are locked in place. You don't try to move toward your wants, needs, or goals—not because you have no goals or don't want anything; rather, perhaps you feel you do not deserve to meet your goals or have the things you want. You may have been let down so many times that the fear of trying again is real. You might not trust positive experiences or feelings, having tolerated negative emotions about yourself and the world for so long. This roadblock keeps you from seeing failures as learning experiences because you might believe you deserve to fail, and this state has become your norm.

I've heard many times that it's hard to handle failure as a member of an immigrant family, because there's also little concept of how to handle success, simply because successes were rarely acknowledged or validated. Hard work and drive were the expected minimums; the only sort of acknowledgment was to ask, "Why didn't you try harder for a loftier goal or accomplishment?" If success came easily, then it wasn't believed to be worth as much. Success seemed to be tied with the need to suffer, and suffering was one way to prove oneself deserving of success. Even more so, success was never celebrated. There might even be a mistrust of praise or celebration because it was so rarely offered. Some children of immigrants may have never witnessed their parents celebrate their own accomplishments and so struggle to do so themselves. We're more likely to punish ourselves for our failures than to recognize all of our gains and growth. Many of us believe that we don't deserve to be recognized for our success and were only "seen" by our parents when we failed. This has created such an imbalance in how we approach failure and success—since we experienced neither positively.

─── REST STOP ───

Do you feel like you don't deserve to succeed? Does this feeling of being undeserving keep you from learning from your failures and facing them with curiosity and compassion instead of criticism and judgment? Do you struggle to acknowledge your success?

A Note on Emotional Responses to Failure

Many of my clients have said, "Can't I just not feel the emotions related to failure? That would be so much easier. Can you help me to just stop feeling?" Does this sound familiar? While it may seem easier, if we were to remove the emotional activation that comes with experiencing shame and failure, we would also remove the emotional salience of these experiences. Emotional salience is a fancy way of identifying how emotionally important or notable an event is in your life. Your wedding day? High emotional salience. Brushing your teeth before bed? Probably pretty low salience. If you did not experience any emotions whenever you failed, you would be much less likely to give it any attention and by extension much less likely to learn from it. Emotions, as we learned in chapter 2, are red flags for important information in our lives. When we experience emotions after failure, it's a tug at our attention saying, "Hey—pay attention to this. There might be something you need to understand, learn, change, or do." So, while you may be able to hold failure and shame more effectively with practice, it will not completely eliminate the emotional hurt or pain that encounters with failure may prompt. This is normal and adaptive.

DISENTANGLING FAILURE FROM SHAME

So, we understand the myths of failure and the roadblocks it presents. How do we move forward? I'm often asked, "How do I learn how to fail?" My answer is the same each time:

1. Get comfortable with discomfort and negative emotion.
2. Name the shame that has been wrapped around the failure.
3. Consider what the failure is bringing to you instead of what it is taking away.
4. Consider what next step you can take with the information failure offers you.
5. Try again through action.

Perhaps it's easier said than done, but I truly believe that when we are able to move through these steps, failure takes on a different shape and meaning. No longer is failure an indication of internal deficits; it's an opportunity to try a new solution or idea. No longer is failure a source of shame; it's a chance to refocus and find a new direction. None of this can happen if we avoid failure and the shame it can trigger. When we are unable to detach our shame from our failures, we will struggle to embrace and move through them, and we will likely get stuck.

If we allow ourselves to face our shame, transform that shame into power, and release it from failure as an identity narrative, failure becomes a pathway to success. We can then gain access to unlimited potential for growth and expansion in our lives. We learn how to engage with ourselves with compassion and kindness rather than harshness and judgment. We develop courage to persist in the face of obstacles toward our goals. We shape our identity as we develop character in the face of defeat and realize that we are someone who will stand back up and keep trying despite the odds. We experience vulnerability that instead of bringing more shame, actually sets us free from it. And we enable connection with others as they receive and hold our failures and vulnerability with empathy. When failure is able to break free from shame, it becomes a powerful tool that helps us build the life we want.

Facing Our Shame

The first step to disentangling failure from shame is recognizing that shame is created in relationships. If we each lived in isolation and never came in contact with others, we would rarely experience shame, because there would be no one to shame us. As we explored in chapter 4, if not for our relationships, if we did something wrong, there would be no one to make fun of us, scold us, or make us feel bad about it. We would just move about our day having made the mistake and learning from it (sometimes) for next time. In reality, we are surrounded by people who are all the time observing, watching, and witnessing parts of our lives, and when they react poorly to our mistakes or failures, the seed of shame is planted.

This disentangling usually begins in relationships with others; when we can meet in a safe space with another individual or individuals and open up about our shame, we have the opportunity to experience compassion offered by others. We can see that what we believed to be so bad, broken, or wrong with us actually is not as bad as we thought. We see that others may also have experienced something similar, and there is a shared humanity that reminds us that there is actually nothing wrong with us after all.

Many times, my clients will share something they have been ashamed about for most of their lives. Often, after they share their deep, dark secret, they will say, "I've never told anyone else this before." And then they will share a deep sense of relief that this secret has finally been brought to light, that it has been seen and witnessed by another person, who has received it without judgment. Speaking our shame is one way we can purge its toxicity and keep it from eroding our self-concept. Think of it as holding our shame in one hand while clutching to compassion with the other. Compassion from others in tandem with self-compassion can reduce or extinguish the flames of shame before they set our identity on fire.

Learning to sit with our shame while not internalizing it is a discipline. It is not instinctual—most of us have been taught to shame ourselves throughout our lives. Working with a therapist can be a powerful way to move through failure and shame. If therapy is not accessible, finding a trusted and safe person to share the shame with can also be helpful. If nothing else, writing about our failure and shame can provide the necessary outlet and distance to begin to reprogram our ideas surrounding shame and failure.

——— REST STOP ———

How have you encountered your feelings of shame in the past? Are there key moments in your life when you experienced shame and tried to avoid it? What stories has that shame told you about yourself and your abilities?

Reframing Failure

When I was growing up, there was no discussion about the benefits of failure. Everything was framed around avoiding failure at all costs—no one was inviting us to fail as a path to success. In recent years, researchers like Carol Dweck and Angela Duckworth have been asking us to question how we think about failure, and reframing failure has become wildly popular in leadership, management, teaching, and mental health.

What conclusions have these discussions led to? First, failure is not bad. In fact, it might be a good thing. It's hard to believe when you've been told your whole life that being a failure was not an option. Instead, current research suggests that we can approach failure with different mindsets, specifically a growth or fixed mindset. This concept is gaining steady popularity and is detailed at length in Dweck's book *Mindset*. Suffice to say, a fixed mindset holds the belief that we all possess specific skills and talents, and no matter how much effort we apply, we can't change that potential, whereas a growth mindset holds we all possess unbounded potential for growth and evolution. Possession of a fixed mindset means any struggle or failure is attributed to one's incapacity for growth. A growth mindset makes the simple act of trying enough to take you on your journey forward, wherein failure is a pitstop where you refuel for your journey forward, allowing you to redirect or refine your approach to a problem.

The way you interpret failure has a significant impact on whether or not you keep showing up and doing the work or whether you shut down and give up. The way we frame failure also impacts the risks and opportunities that we might take to get the things we want in our lives. The scarcity mentality we discussed previously (see chapter 1) can creep up here, too; if you believe that there are not enough opportunities or resources out there for you, then taking a risk or making a mistake can feel like a huge risk. The reality is that most people, once they find the courage to make a change, are grateful they found the resolve to move forward rather than to stay in the same unhappy place.

⟞ REST STOP ⟞

How do you currently frame failure? Do you tend to operate from a fixed or growth mindset? How has this mindset served you? How has this mindset limited you? What new opportunity or thing would you try if you reframed your mindset on failure?

THE BEAUTY OF WHOLEHEARTED TRYING

By now, you know that we can think all day, but without action, it is unlikely that our lives will change. When we have begun the work of detangling our failure from shame, we need to start moving our muscles and trying new things. Action is the way in which we gain the data necessary to move through failure. Perhaps you're thinking you're too scared (and scarred) from your past failures to act. Here, I encourage you to take the next small step.

So many times when we are trying to act, we get scared, and our fight-or-flight response comes online. Then we start telling ourselves we must aim for this huge goal, and we must do it all today, and when we don't hit the huge goal and get it all done today, we say, "Yep. See I knew it. I am a failure." In this scenario, you quite literally set yourself up for failure. When we try new and scary things, we need to find the fine balance between taking tangible steps and overwhelming our nervous systems so much that we just shut down.

A Good College Try

The semester I discovered psychology, I was insatiable. I often trolled Half Price Books on the weekends looking for any textbooks or resources on psychology topics. It was the first time in my life that I was truly interested in a field of study. Over the summer, I read through as many books as I could find on various psychological conditions and theories of attachment and personality—and not because I was preparing for any test or coursework. I truly found it stimulating and exciting to immerse myself in the topic. This is when I knew I had stumbled upon something special, something important that was worth walking away from my established career path. Prior to this point, education was a chore; I had to participate in it in order to get to something else. I had never truly tasted what it was like to learn for pleasure and joy. I had never tapped into this form of clean energy and motivation before. When moving through failure, look for the spark. That's often where we can tap into clean energy sources for the journey. Following are some techniques that are helpful when trying to move forward in action in spite of our fears of failure.

One of the most important things we can do when working through previous failures is to identify our goal and break it down to achievable, tangible steps—you may be familiar with the idea of SMART goals (specific, measurable, achievable, realistic, and time-bound). This turns our goals into stepping-stones instead of a journey up Everest and reduces avoidance or procrastination, which can come on quite strong when we try to move past our failures. To start, your plan can be three simple, tangible steps you can take immediately.

Next, check in with your body and mind and assess safety. Ask yourself if there's anything you can add to your efforts or to a situation to make it feel safer. Safety can be built by accessing more information, recruiting social support, and practicing skills. Talk to someone who has been there before you; chat with a friend to process your thoughts. Creating safety is necessary to protect yourself and your nervous system so that you are much more likely to follow through instead of making up excuses or procrastinating.

Finally, check in with your curiosity. The thought of trying again or doing something new can be quite triggering and overwhelm the nervous system. To push past this, I encourage you to seek out sparks of curiosity, excitement, or interest. In *Grit*, Angela Duckworth discusses how interests and passion are two building blocks for perseverance and grit. Where we have previously been motivated by avoiding failure, it's now necessary to find other types of motivation. A client offered a beautiful insight, which I'll share with you here: Fear-based motivation is like fossil fuels—they get the engine running, but they burn dirty. These fossil fuels make us doubt ourselves and question our abilities; they power that little voice of self-doubt we all have. Clean energy, which can be found in spaces of curiosity, passion, meaning, and purpose, can also move us toward our goals while leaving our identity and self-esteem intact. We can employ interest, passion, connection, and excitement as the fuel for our important work. Burning clean energy gives us motivation to act and move toward our goals without setting our mental health on fire to burn as motivation.

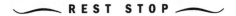

REST STOP

Can you tell when you are burning fossil fuels versus clean energy to move toward your goals? How do you feel when you are burning these two types of energy? Which energy source empowers and excites you? What might burning clean energy look like for you?

MOVING THROUGH FAILURE

In this exercise, you will practice how to move through failure instead of getting stuck in it. I encourage you to think about a current situation in which you believe you have failed. Use the following stepping-stones to work through the shame, reframe failure, and move toward wholehearted trying. The more you work through these steps, the easier the process will be and the more fluidly you will move through future encounters with failure.

Facing Our Shame:

    How has this experience woven shame stories into your identity?

    Have you ever shared this experience of shame with anyone? Has it ever been held in compassion by another safe person?

    Who might be a safe person who could hold your shame?

    What did it feel like to be able to speak your shame out loud?

    What did this conversation release you from?

Reframing Failure:

    How might you reframe this failure in light of the growth mindset?

    In what ways are you tempted to focus on a fixed mindset for this experience?

    Is the fixed mindset useful in moving you toward your goals?

    What is possible if you were to reframe this failure from a growth mindset?

The Beauty of Trying:

    What is your ideal goal?

    Break down your ideal goal into small, achievable, and tangible steps.

    Break them down even further (I see you trying to bite off a huge piece).

    Do you notice a spark anywhere in that goal of yours? What is the spark?

    As you embark on action to move through failure, what kind of energy are you motivated by? Clean energy or fossil fuels?

    Which energy source feels more sustainable and compassionate?

Bonus Step—Evaluate Feedback from Actions:

    What happened after you took a small, tangible action?

    What kind of feedback did you receive?

What was useful and helpful feedback?

How can you integrate that feedback for your next small tangible action?

Use this exercise whenever you need to process a failure or setback. Eventually, you'll be able to do this naturally, but first, you have to practice.

*   *   *

As we end this leg of our journey, I hope you understand that failure is not what defines you; instead, it is a tool you can access if you can tolerate the discomfort it triggers. But to use failure as a tool instead of a roadblock, you must invest in the work of unlearning the cultural and societal programming you might have received. You must keep yourself from reading failure as evidence of your flaws or deficiencies. You must let go of the stories of needing to be perfect or being not good enough. You must learn to embrace feedback as a gift rather than as criticism of your value and worth. You can use failure to hone your skills, understand your obstacles, and realize you have it within yourself to stand back up and keep pushing. When you find the courage and support to face your fears of failure, you will realize you are capable of things you never imagined. Although the sting of failure may rattle you and cause you to doubt yourself temporarily, it is the way you brush yourself off and decide to still show up and try that really determines whether you have failed or not. All you need to do is try.

CHAPTER 8

Permission to Play

Play is an activity enjoyed for its own sake. It is our brain's favorite way of learning and maneuvering.

—Diane Ackerman

Play is the highest form of research.

—Albert Einstein

When I was a kid, it always felt like there was a fun meter in our household, an imaginary dial that showed how much fun I was allowed to have for the following week. Every Sunday night, the dial would reset itself. If on Monday I asked for a playdate or something fun, I knew for sure that by Friday, the dial would be turned down and any requests for play at the end of the week would receive a resounding "no." The reason for this? If I had time to play, then I didn't have enough work to do. "Go find some work to do before we catch you thinking about playing," my parents would say. The fun meter was so heavily regulated that I had to devise ways to circumvent it. In my middle school years, this often involved making up "school projects" that I needed to work on with friends. Past the age of nine, these were my most frequent memories of play. Play was discouraged. Play was indulgent. Play was irresponsible. Play was a waste of time and took away from the more serious stuff of life.

Having children of my own inspired me to question my assumptions about play. After my graduate training, my postdoctoral fellowship, and hustling to get my private practice running, the decision to hit pause on my career activated all my old narratives about play and self-worth. Up until that point, my worth was heavily tied up in my degree, my achievements, and where my career was headed. After fighting so hard to become a psychologist, I was intentionally hitting the pause button and stepping away from my career to focus on motherhood. I did not realize how difficult of a shift this would be. Suddenly, I was at home for hours at a time watching my daughter play, engaging in the very act that I had disparaged and devalued for a significant portion of my life. Witnessing her exploration, experimentation, and playing for hours shifted my own feelings about play. I realized how much shame had been internalized about my desires to play and how strictly I controlled my ability to play and rest in my adult life. My daughter also made me realize that the enjoyment found within play was worthy enough of being a goal in itself. In fact, it was vital for her development, learning, and experience of boundless joy. It made me wonder what I was losing out on by restricting and limiting play for most of my life.

I share this with you to emphasize how deeply embedded my assumptions about play were and, truthfully, sometimes still are. When my daughter was in second grade, I found her and her brother playing and laughing hysterically at something. Instead of extending curiosity and wondering what they were playing and laughing about, the first thing that came out of my mouth was "Have you finished your homework yet?" Deflated, my kids stopped giggling and looked away in disappointment that their

fun had been interrupted. My partner, who observed the interaction, gently said to me, "Wow. It was almost like they were having
too much fun, and you were not okay with it." I was crushed and
reminded of how instinctual it is for me to believe that play is not
a worthwhile activity. We may instinctually try to stamp it out of
our children—and even more often, stamp it out of ourselves.

It is natural for play to be more enjoyable than work; setting
healthy boundaries around work and play gives us space for both.
As adults, more often than not, we struggle less with playing too
much—play without limits can be problematic—and more with
lack of any play at all in our lives. We struggle with our inability to
move flexibly and compassionately through seasons of work and
play without guilt or shame. It's not your fault that you struggle
with play, but it is now your responsibility to reprogram your relationship with it. Play is so important that ignoring it or putting
it off can lead to burnout. Play allows you to keep in touch with
yourself and helps guide you along your journey of self-discovery.
Allowing yourself the freedom to play makes it possible for you to
access moments of joy and connection.

As we enter this chapter, I invite you into the eighth leg of our
journey: giving yourself permission to play. Play is the birthplace
of exploration, experimentation, and mindful presence. Perhaps
you're thinking, *This is unrealistic—I'm an adult; I don't have
time to play.* I invite you to think about play not always as a specific act or time set aside, but perhaps as a posture or way of living our lives, being attuned to our energy and mindset, and, when
possible, inviting play in, no matter how mundane of a task we
are doing. My daughter still reminds me of the time we had a mini
rave in our living room after she found a stash of glow sticks;
we danced to music until we were out of breath. Something as
simple as cooking dinner can be a burden or an opportunity for

connection or mindful nourishment. Opportunities for play are all around us, but we often miss them in our distracted, busy, and overwhelmed states. What are we all working so hard for if not to obtain joy, play, and ease? If we have the power to choose how we see these precious few moments of our lives, will your moments be rainbows or roadblocks? I hope you choose rainbows when you can. I hope you choose to play and give yourself a chance to find the magic.

⟍— REST STOP —⟋

What is your relationship with the idea of play? What narratives become activated when you consider playing? How does your body feel when you are in play? Does it seize up, or does it melt into the rhythm of not having to produce? Can you move fluidly through work and play, or do you get stuck in a certain zone?

UNTRUE STORIES ABOUT PLAY

From a biological perspective, it is almost impossible to engage in play when we are under threat. In previous chapters, we discussed the two branches of the autonomic nervous system: sympathetic and parasympathetic. The sympathetic nervous system is what powers our fight-or-flight mode in response to real or perceived danger. This inhibits parasympathetic nervous system activity, which includes rest, restoration, exploration, and play.

Let's now consider how many of our parents came to the United States with survival as the primary goal. Some came with only a few dollars in their pocket, while others might have come with resources but arrived alone and unable to speak the language. Any of these scenarios could activate the sympathetic nervous system. For our forebears, the act of work became their ticket to safety and security, and in pursuit of this safety and security, they gave up the ability to rest or take a day off. There was no opportunity to prioritize play—in survival and scarcity mode, play drops off first, postponed until we feel safe. Postponing play is adaptive for survival. It allows all our most useful resources to be channeled toward solving the problem ahead of us or evading threat. What happens if we never feel safe and are stuck in survival mentality? Many of us continue to carry the legacy of this burden, handed over from our parents' stories and experiences. How many of us witnessed our parents working seven days a week, putting off rest and play for many years, and sacrificing physical and mental health in the process? How many of us have internalized certain ideas around rest and play? We may have learned that play is not necessary, that there are better things to do, and that devoting time to play can get in the way of our goals. We have learned that play is silly, child-like, or lazy. A particularly strong narrative is that rest and play are only to be had once they've been earned with work. If you haven't earned it, then you do not deserve it. As a result, playing can induce a tremendous amount of guilt. These strong emotional reactions of hypercriticism or guilt often stand in the way of us accessing play as a natural and necessary part of our lives.

All of this stems from the stories we have been told about play over the course of our lives. At some point, play moved from being acceptable to being unacceptable—from being appropriate when we are children to being shameful now that we are adults. Let's explore some of these frameworks together. I encourage you to consider which of these you might hold for the concept of play, and to gently challenge and question for yourself whether these frameworks are truly serving you.

Play Is a Waste

Play exists only for itself and the enjoyment of it—it has no ulterior motive or goal. This puts it in strong opposition to survival mentality. It's why so many of our parents cautioned us when we took too many days of vacation or shamed us for enjoying life too much—from a survival mentality, play is considered to be a waste of time and energy that should be devoted to a higher goal or outcome, such as ambition, advancement, or financial wealth. Play says it is okay to reclaim the minutes of our lives instead of wasting them through numbed distraction and disconnected consumerism, disrupting the obsessive striving our society feeds off of in order to maintain the capitalist structures that keep people in jobs they don't love and buying things they don't need. This makes it potentially dangerous for our mental health.

Those who struggle with play view it as especially wasteful. It is something they long for so much but rarely allow themselves to taste, and so they become upset when others engage in it. Witnessing someone allowing themselves to play may breed resentment; they may think, *Why can they play, but I can't?* Play can also create fear, in the sense that we may get so wrapped up in the feelings of nourishment and connection when we allow ourselves to play that we fear we won't want to return to working hard or achieving our goals.

—— **REST STOP** ——

When was the last time that you played without judging yourself? When you engage in rest and play, what kind of self-talk rises to the surface?

Play Is Selfish and Childlike

Play is commonly considered an act only for children, so much so that adults are often shamed or ridiculed when we engage in play. In your older adolescent years, did you frequently hear statements like "Stop acting like a child" or "Will you just grow up"? When adults are unable to handle or manage their responsibilities, children may unknowingly shoulder the burdens of this overflow in responsibility, essentially becoming parentified children. Some children of immigrants were latchkey kids who came back from school to empty homes because their parents were working long hours. Others were expected to take care of younger siblings— even making sure they did their homework and chores. Some of us might have acted like marriage and family therapists, often having to mediate between parents as they fought through difficult conflicts. Many clients have shared that they felt as though they never had a chance to experience a "normal" childhood, one in which they could just be kids, not responsible for other family members or filling gaps their parents couldn't. Play can also feel selfish—if you have work, family, and commitments, of course you won't want to let those who depend on you down by taking time to enjoy yourself. Practicing play may fill you with immense guilt, as though you're somehow putting off what others expect of you. I see this especially in parents who juggle multiple careers and family responsibilities. They rarely allow themselves even an hour a week to step away from all responsibilities to rest or play.

Play is a learned behavior. If most of your childhood was filled with moments when you were scolded for playing, shamed for wasting time, and asked to shoulder adult responsibilities, then your struggle to engage in play as an adult should come as no surprise. It's likely that few of us had this behavior modeled for us by the adults in our lives—perhaps our parents didn't participate in any hobbies or interests that had no tangible value aside from pleasure or enjoyment. So how could we know that play is healthy, normal, and necessary?

──── R E S T S T O P ────

Who, if anyone, modeled play for you? Did you witness your parents or important adults in your life giving themselves permission to play? If not, what would that have looked like, and what would it have meant to you to witness it?

Play Interrupts Productivity

It should come as no surprise that a number of the adults I work with struggle to play, because their to-do list is a mile long. When time and energy are finite resources, the act of play can seem frivolous at best and foolish at worst. Some of my clients can barely find time to eat and feel immense guilt for neglecting their children and relationships; when we discuss play, they look at me like I've grown antlers. My response to this usually is "So, when will you ever get to notice your life? Notice the people? Notice the emotions? Notice the joy? When do you actually get to the living part of life instead of doing?"

The reality is that your to-do list will always exist. Everything else is changeable: Kids grow up, partners become neglected and frustrated, health problems don't wait for you to be less busy before demanding attention. What are you missing out on by avoiding play? The smell of coffee that your partner makes for you during a fall morning. Your child's laugh as you read them their favorite book. The feeling of flow when you are focused on a hobby that resets your mind. Play is the *fuel* for your productivity, not a detractor. Play offers you the rest and spark to return to the things you care about and that are worthy of your time. It gets you ready for the climb toward your next goal.

Instead, we put off rest and play until we have "more time," and eventually the consequences of our neglect catch up with us— physical or emotional breakdowns, broken relationships (romantic and otherwise), career disappointments. My intent isn't to be a fearmonger; my hope for you is that you won't have to experience one of these wake-up calls in order to get clear on what you care about most in your life. Play encourages us to be aware, to slow down a bit and notice how we actually feel about our lives and what is happening within them.

REST STOP

Are you fully conscious and aware of the life that you are living? Or do you feel like you are going through the motions and feeling dissociated from both the good and the bad parts of your life? Can you remember the last time you truly engaged in rest and play?

Play as Medicine

While play can provide space for new beginnings and exploration, it can also give us the chance to be reminded of our "why" and gain perspective in the midst of the muck and messiness of life. While writing this book, I experienced one of the most intense seasons of burnout in my life. The convergence of world events that deeply affected me— George Floyd's murder; the massacre of Asian spa workers in Atlanta—coupled with the steadily increasing exhaustion and worry from the COVID-19 pandemic sent me into a tailspin, physically and mentally. Of course, I couldn't have anticipated all these life events—and all of them left me burned to a crisp.

So, I did what felt like the most counterproductive thing I could do, as deadlines loomed: I booked a trip to visit college friends for a weekend in San Diego. It felt like I was digging myself into a deeper hole, but I needed to find my way back to myself again. I was having serious doubts—about writing, about my work—and I wondered if I should just call everything off and go back to focusing on the more regular parts of my life. While packing, it took every ounce of willpower to leave my laptop at home, ignoring the voice in my head telling me that my time on the flight would give me ample opportunity to write. I brought a novel instead. I forced my body to rest and invited myself into play. During dinner one night, fully present for the first time in months, I burst into tears and said, "This might be the first time I am enjoying food in a really long time." I had run myself ragged, and at that moment I fully realized how tattered I had become. I had lived with such strong blinders that I had forgotten how to enjoy and savor food and my life. This thought was extremely depressing. My friends held me in love and nonjudgment for the whole weekend. They reminded me of who I was, of why I was writing this book, and that I was capable of it. It was exactly what I needed—a necessary pause and permission to play without having earned a thing.

Whatever your life circumstances, can you find the time to allow yourself to consider how you might introduce play as a healing practice for exhaustion and as a form of medicine for our epidemic of over-functioning, loneliness, and burnout? Perhaps for you this medicine may come in the form of planning dinner and a movie at home with your kids, where you put away your phones and just savor the evening, or taking an hour out of your day to go for a leisurely walk with a friend and notice every smell of fall in the air. Play does not have to be a lavish trip to an exotic location; it can be found in the ordinary moments, if you are willing to create magic within every day.

THE GIFTS OF PLAY

A particularly sad part of adulthood is that we adopt all these rules for living that aren't actually our own. These rules keep society flowing efficiently and productively, but they seldom help us live life well. If we can intentionally unlearn these rules and shake off a little of the hold they have on us, we can gain access to the gifts of play. We can take advantage of the richness that comes from safe spaces to explore and be curious about this life and the potential of realizing that each day is a gift instead of a burden. We can experience the connection of being present with those in our lives who seek only our presence and attention. Play offers us a glimpse into parts of our lives that we are too busy to notice when we are in the grind of life.

In my own life, I have had to learn how to move more fluidly through a season of intense work, such as when I was in graduate school juggling my dissertation, clinical work, and moonlighting for extra cash in the psychiatric emergency room and not prioritizing times of rest and play. The truth is that avoiding play was a way to cope with my anxiety and feelings of not being enough. If I slowed down or paused—if I played—it would force me to confront the parts of myself I knew were not happy with my over-functioning all the time. Avoiding play made it possible for me to keep those parts of myself at bay and ignore all the warning signs that perhaps I needed to make changes in my life.

I now consider moments of play like oases along life's journey. Sometimes these oases appear by accident, and other times we chart our course in search of them so that we can finally set down our luggage, find a comforting place to eat, and look around to marvel at how far we have come. In Paulo Coelho's *The Alchemist*, the main character stumbles upon an oasis, and there he meets a person he has been searching for his entire life. Had he not taken a pit stop at the oasis, he never would have found her. Sometimes we believe that the things we are searching for happen only when we are striving for them. Instead, sometimes those things are right in front of us, but we cannot see them because we are so distracted by the striving itself.

If it feels right, pause here and consider why play may be such a struggle for you. If it's not, reflect on that instead. However, if you have a hard time engaging in play, could you be open to the idea that play isn't necessarily a waste, selfish, childish, or unproductive? Perhaps you are now challenging the way you live because the way you've been doing it has not brought you fulfillment, happiness, or joy. Below, I share with you some of the gifts of play I and those I work with received when we began to invite play into our

lives. These are just some examples, and I encourage you to consider what play has brought you over the course of your life. What
has the act of play allowed you to access and invited you into?
If play hasn't been a priority for you, could you consider creating more of these experiences in your life and see what is revealed
within you?

Play Is the Birthplace of Creativity and Exploration

When we play, we are engaged in the active space of focused attention and curiosity. It demands our full attention, as we notice new
sensations or explore novel ideas. Within play we have both the
safety and freedom to think outside of the box, experiment, and
try new combinations that otherwise would not be possible in the
"real world." Play creates a space that suspends reality, rules, and
expectations, allowing our minds to fill in the gaps and create
new connections. Play combats the pessimistic, critical, and rule-
based thinking that we have internalized from the outside world,
making space for us to dream and hope in the potential of infinite
opportunities.

There's a reason play makes us feel good. In this state of enjoyment and immersion, our parasympathetic nervous system acts to
calm us and helps us connect with others in a more vulnerable
and authentic way. We feel safer sharing ideas with others, even
the outlandish, outside-of-the-box ones. It generates the spark we
discussed in previous chapters, the kindling for new passions and
interests. It also allows us to access an inner resilience that believes
in infinite possibilities versus scarcity and fear.

⌣⌢ R E S T   S T O P ⌢⌣

When was the last time you had a chance to play? What kind of play feels good for you? Can you access the mindset of play you had as a child? What is it trying to tell you?

Play Encourages Presence

As I mentioned earlier, play has no ulterior motive. If it did, it would lose its magic. Play cannot thrive under striving or pressure. It shrinks in the face of anxiety or future-oriented thinking. Play depends on your ability to stay in the here and now, which is why play and rest can feel so elusive. In our current age, we are all struggling to stay present. We're met with a lot of anxiety-provoking information and experiences—it's hard to participate in social media, for example, without feeling like the world is falling apart. Because of this, it's important that we let ourselves surrender to play and gently draw our attention to the present, to breathe in the moment, to tune into our bodies and minds right here and now. That is when play and rest can thrive. Play, at its very essence, encourages us to be present. It gently says, "Notice. Look around you. What do you see, feel, hear, taste, and experience?"

More than one of my clients has shared their struggle to understand how to rest and play. They unwind by binge-watching Netflix or they zone out on their phones, doomscrolling their way into the early hours of the morning. I often have to remind them of the difference between rest and dissociation. Rest is restorative and replenishing while we remain fully present, and it connects us more deeply to our current experience. Dissociation, on the other hand, is a form of avoidance that disconnects us from the present moment and intentional awareness. It distracts rather than restores. It numbs our senses and dulls our minds instead of making us more attuned and aware of our current experience. So, the question is, When you rest, are you truly resting, or are you dissociating from your life in order to numb the negative feelings?

⟋⟋⟋ REST STOP ⟋⟋⟋

Think about your recent moments of rest. Do they feel restful or restless? What types of behaviors do you practice in order to rest? How effective are they in helping you access your rest? When you play, do you feel disconnected or reconnected to your current experience?

Play Affirms Inherent Worth

The act of play can be a revolutionary act of allowing ourselves, as children of immigrants, freedom from harshness and criticism. When we give ourselves permission to rest and play, we are expressing to others and ourselves that we deserve that right as a human being. We do not need to earn it, proving our worth through productivity. The opportunity to play belongs to us as much as it belongs to others.

This feeling of needing to earn rest or play can be difficult to unlearn. Many of the people I work with describe an inherent feeling of unworthiness when it comes to playfulness and restfulness. As we discussed at the beginning of the chapter, without positive models, the message becomes that value comes from obedience and achievement. Instead of feeling inherent worth, the feeling is that relationships are transactional in nature—one A+ gaining you a brief moment of rest, a short-term reprieve from having to produce. But these moments are fleeting and must be earned over and over again.

Many clients also have shared that they received very little parental warmth or physical or verbal affection as children. While this is not unusual within Asian cultures, the lack of spontaneous affection only served to reinforce the tit-for-tat nature of our earliest relationships. As a new generation, we need to change this. When I hug my children randomly in the middle of our day, they have not had to do a single thing to earn it. I am offering it because my child has value to me that extends beyond anything they can "do" to earn it. When we rarely experience acts of love, warmth, or positive affection from our parents except when they are dangled on the end of a stick, it can feel as though we don't deserve that love unless we have something to show for it. There is no intent here to blame or condemn our parents—they likely never experienced this type of love themselves and couldn't access ideas or behaviors they had never known. They, too, unwittingly participated in this cycle.

REST STOP

Do you struggle with deserving rest irrespective of your effort or work? What do you believe you need to do in order to deserve your rest or play? Why do you think you use rest as a reward for good behavior rather than fuel for pursuing your goals? Who taught you to relate to play and rest in this way?

CULTIVATING PLAY

In my clinical work, the theme of play eventually emerges once my clients have had a chance to address the fires and crises of their lives, when they feel safe and secure and no longer in a state of fight or flight, having moved through the intense emotionality of discontent, unhappiness, or depression. As these areas of their lives improve, they have more capacity to open up and allow themselves to experience the gifts of play. This is not to say that we must wait until we are in a perfectly calm or fully regulated state in order to play, but play can be quite difficult when we are under distress. I share these suggestions for cultivating play spaces to support your exploration of play through a fresh pair of eyes. I encourage you to consider how you might integrate these concepts as you relearn how to play again. Once you start, your inner child will lead you the rest of the way back to your playful, loved, and cherished self.

Follow the Body

The body does not lie. You cannot fake the sensation of true pleasure. You cannot trick your body into believing that you are safe. The body knows what it feels, and it feels what it feels for a reason. The body does not easily bypass its feelings or reactions quite like the mind is sometimes capable of doing. The body is much harder to distract from or gaslight when it is feeling overwhelmed. With this in mind, I encourage you to tune into your body. How does it feel at the end of a long day? Instead of numbing yourself with mindless scrolling or endless TV, take a moment and be still. Listen to your body and how it is reacting to the here and now. When was the last time your body felt at ease? When was the last time it played?

The body can forget what it is like to play. This is why novelty, travel, and unique experiences can keep our playfulness alive. In a new setting and under a new context, we feel less bound by the rigid rules of our day-to-day routines. We are also more inspired to try new things. Play in the body can be a full range of experiences. It can be taste, touch, smell, warmth, connection, swaying, rhythms, and so many sensations and experiences in between. If it has been a long time since you have experienced play in your body, start by just turning on some music in the privacy of your room. Close your eyes and give your body permission to react as it wants to, be it nodding, swaying, twirling, or humming. Do whatever the body feels led to do without hesitation or limitation. If your mind wanders to a space of worry or distraction while your body is moving, draw your attention back into your body with gentleness and kindness. When we struggle with play, we often also struggle with bodily presence too. This is normal. As you ease your body back into the space of play, you may find that it becomes easier and easier to remain present in the play and that the mind will wander less.

───── **REST STOP** ─────

How is your body feeling right now? When you give yourself a moment to tune in, what do you notice? Is there something that your body might be needing or craving right now? What kind of rest or play might your body enjoy at this moment? How might you best meet that need in your body?

Play as the End Goal

Play is only concerned with enjoyment, not outcome. As you begin the process of relearning how to play, it is important to remember that play is not meant to lead you anywhere except for here and back into yourself and others. We often feel temptation to take something we love, some part of our play, and try to convert it into something that has an end goal or function. We feel the need to hustle, to capitalize on and monetize our play, which takes anything we remotely enjoy for fun and turns it into work. I am not discouraging this entirely—in several cases, doing something you love that you also find fun can become your livelihood. What I want you to do is to deeply consider how your relationship with this fun activity or hobby might change once it becomes an opportunity. Research suggests that once our motivation for a certain behavior moves from internal or intrinsic motivation (interest, curiosity, passion) to an external or extrinsic motivation (money, status, fame), we start to experience a decline in our subjective enjoyment of it.

While it can be a great way to keep in contact with others, learn, and find like-minded people, social media has become a driving force in our lives, and as we might feel drawn to document, post, and share our play, the enjoyment of it becomes secondary. We've all chuckled at a table of restaurant guests obsessively photographing their food (the camera eats first), and we have all likely done that at one point or another. In this way, play becomes a way for us to showcase our lives and compare ourselves to others. When we focus more on the documentation of play over the actual act of play and rest, we have lost some of the point. Whenever I feel the tug to look at my phone while spending time with others, or to post photos of my kids, I try to reground myself by asking, "If I didn't take a picture or video of this moment, would I still enjoy it?" Our phones have become ubiquitous, but it's okay to put them down for a while and play. Perhaps we can encourage each other to use social media as a tool to add to the richness of our lives instead of keeping us from being able to remain present in them.

—— REST STOP ——

What activities do you enjoy doing that are focused only on enjoyment, pleasure, and joy as the outcome? How often do you engage in these activities? What emotions do you experience when you are in these activities? What keeps you from doing these activities more often?

Plan Your Play

The idea of scheduling play seems like an oxymoron. Surely, play should be spontaneous and unstructured, right? That may be the case, if you are a child, or an adult who happens to have fewer distractions or obligations. However, most of us have many responsibilities grabbing for attention every day. As much as I would like to believe that we can all be self-motivated enough to play spontaneously and unexpectedly, the reality is that we tend to default to our natural state, usually one of fulfilling expectations or playing out the different roles that society has set for us or that we have set. It can be hard after so many years of functioning without play and rest to suddenly shift gears and expect to move fluidly between work and play with ease.

So, as strange as it may sound, cultivating play is a discipline. It's something that must be practiced over and over. It must be prioritized and scheduled so that we engage in play at a regular cadence, not just when we get so burned out that we feel compelled to book a last-minute vacation to escape our intense lifestyle, or when we become so sick that we're forced to take sick days because our bodies have nothing left to give. We can't wait for things to get bad for us to play, so intentionally making the time allows us to use play as the fuel for getting through life's difficulties instead of being an escape hatch. Play and rest shouldn't be reactive. Scheduling play is like preventative medicine, done in order to help replenish and be better able to focus on what matters most to you. Find what you enjoy doing and try as much as possible to schedule time for it.

What is a play-based activity that you have been wanting to add into your life? Is it for you alone, or are there others you want to get involved? What is preventing you from scheduling this activity on your calendar? How might you turn this into a more consistent gathering or space for yourself and perhaps others? What might this recurring event bring to your life?

GO PLAY

In lieu of a formal exercise, I urge you to get up and *play*. Start small, and then build up. Schedule it. Do it without guilt or regret. I hope you've had a chance to explore how you relate to the concept of play and can see with more clarity the different rules and expectations that may have been placed upon you that kept you from being able to play with safety and freedom. If you need it, let the process of relearning how to play help you get past any historical fears you may have been exposed to—ones that kept you from playing without having to earn the opportunity first. Growing up as children of immigrants, we may have learned to live through a posture of self-denial—of pleasure, enjoyment, leisure, or joy. Participating in play rejects self-denial. Giving ourselves permission to play and rest reminds us that we are beloved and inherently worthy. Play presents the opportunity to fill in gaps our parents or caregivers may have left in our upbringing, and it lets us feel loved without any strings attached, without distraction or transaction. When we struggle with play, it is often because we feel that we do not deserve it. But we do deserve it. Let's put play first as the fuel for our important and hard work in relationships, in careers, and in our lives. Let's just get out there and *play*.

CHAPTER 9

Permission to Grieve

Give sorrow words: The grief that does not speak
Whispers the o'er-fraught heart and bids it break.
—WILLIAM SHAKESPEARE, *MACBETH*

You cannot prevent the birds of sorrow from flying over your
head, but you can prevent them from building nests in your hair.
—CHINESE PROVERB

I miss my ah gong (阿公), my grandfather. I wish I could have seen him one last time and that he could have met his grandchildren, Evie and Theo—they would have made him smile. They would have held his wrinkled hand, and he would have seen how his life touched theirs.

My ah gong connected all of us to those who came before. He allowed me to truly be a child when the world demanded that I grow up. I can still see him, reading his Bible in the morning, the sunlight hitting his face just so as he prayed in the quiet. He seemed to have unyielding patience, withstanding the noise and chaos all around, remaining grounded in himself and his faith. I wish I had had many more years with him; I regret the things that we didn't have time for. I know I will see him once again someday.

THE THIRD SPACE

It always surprises me how your heart can suffer over the loss of someone you barely knew, or how you can long for a land that you cannot call home, or how we search for a sense of belonging and find ourselves disappointed again and again. My story of grief, as a person of scattered origins, somehow always returns back to my maternal grandfather, Chen Ming Shin, which translates to "a life of faith." He was there when we boarded the plane for America for the first time. He was the one I returned to Taiwan to see. A man of few words, he possessed a warm and grounded spirit, and he represents to me all that I love about Taiwan and also all that breaks my heart about my migration journey.

As members of Asian diasporas, we are separated from our native lands. Some of us may remember the places our ancestors called home, while others may have no memories of any such place. Whether we are immigrants or adoptees or know only the land our families emigrated to, it can feel as though we are lost and roaming the earth, searching for a place to take root, only to find that no such place exists. A fellow mental health clinician who is also a transracial Asian adoptee described living in a "third space." I have long felt this third space—a space between worlds and within margins. It is within this third space that we experience many known and unknown losses as children of immigrants or adoptees. It is not just a loss of people or places, but of experiences, memories, and a life that we could have lived had we not made our migration journey. We may grieve the life that could have been, in which we could be more grounded and rooted in our ancestry. The tragic part is that the losses of diasporic peoples do not diminish with time but might actually amplify as life progresses.

By this I mean that as we journey through life searching for a home, we are constantly reminded that our home may not be a place we can locate on a map, but rather a space that we must create for ourselves. Many of us may not have fully realized that we have suffered from loss as people living outside our native lands. Perhaps we felt sadness but couldn't name it. Many of our losses go unnamed and unacknowledged—but grief doesn't disappear, even when it goes unacknowledged or is disavowed. Instead, when we are unable to name our spaces of grief, we push them outside of our conscious awareness to a space where the pain lingers but does not heal. The grief becomes frozen and compartmentalized. It drives a wedge within us, and between us and our people. And as a result, we become cut off from the very parts of ourselves that we are often searching for the most.

As this ninth leg of our journey begins, I invite you to give yourself the permission to grieve. This is the part of our journey in which we might allow ourselves to break just a bit, to soften for just a moment, and to name the heartbreak that it is to live as a scattered people, to be a person with a home but perhaps no homeland, to be seen as a foreigner in our own ancestral lands, and to be reminded that we are outsiders in countries of migration. I've asked myself many times, "How do I move forward from this place of loss?" What I have learned is that we cannot move forward without fully witnessing, naming, and speaking our losses. Though we may try to bypass the grief of migration, there is always a price to pay for unprocessed grief. This is why this part of our journey requires us to remember, search, and excavate our stories, as these acts validate the grief we have felt for perhaps our entire lives, but could not name. When we acknowledge what we have lost, we begin moving into spaces of inner knowing and freedom.

—~ R E S T   S T O P ~—

As a person living outside of your ancestors' homeland, what losses can you name and acknowledge? Are there spaces in which your heart aches, but you are uncertain as to why? What longing, grief, and mourning exist in that third space?

PATHWAYS OF LOSS

People of Asian diasporas have been making their journeys across seas for centuries, and the story of how each of us arrived on distant shores shapes our migration loss in unimaginable ways. The pathways of loss are varied and unique—much like the grief that follows. Our migration journeys span from recent years to several generations past. They are made with smooth and secure passage or fraught with danger, trauma, and poverty. Sometimes the journey was made by choice; others traveled without giving their consent. The story of this first journey can be a source of pain or reflect the hope for opportunities. While I am unable to capture all of the pathways of loss for all Asian diasporas, these are a few common pathways that have emerged personally and in my clinical practice. I encourage you to think about your own and your family's journey. What stories have been wrapped around that migration journey? What was shared with you about the trek? What was hidden from your knowledge? What remains unspoken about your or your parents' migration journey?

Loss through Departure and Separation

One of the most painful sources of grief is the loss caused by physical separation from the people and places of our origin. First- and

1.5-generation immigrants—those who were born in another country and immigrated as children or young adults—may feel this deeply, recalling tearful goodbyes with aunts, uncles, grandparents, and cousins, and missing homemade meals that evoke nostalgia of another lifetime. Second- and third-generation immigrants, those who were born outside of their country of origin, may also feel this if they have visited their homelands and felt the pain of leaving extended family after each trip. This grief can also be experienced among Asian adoptees who had a birth family they left behind, often without a choice. Some of us may remember these journeys through photos, mementos, or even vivid memories of our lives prior to leaving our homeland. In our most profound moments of isolation in our new countries, we can feel so much grief over a community that might exist somewhere faraway but that we cannot access.

For more recent immigrants, those who immigrate in adulthood for school, work, or marriage, the loss of intimate family ties is even more profound as they try to create lives in new countries. Yet, they may feel pulled to relationships and responsibilities in their homelands, a push and pull that's constantly on their minds. A client recently reflected upon his grief as he shared his culture's practice of burying their deceased by sundown on the day of the passing. He lamented that it would be impossible for him to travel back to Asia in time to attend the funeral. The loss of separation is often one of the primary pathways of grief for diasporic communities.

I recall that every few years there would be a long-distance phone call from Taiwan about a relative or family member who was ill or had passed. Each of these times, my parents, stricken in their grief, felt trapped, unable to mobilize the time or finances to make the expensive journey home to attend a funeral or sit bedside with a sick family member. When my grandfather passed, we were told by our extended family not to return. In these subtle ways, we become shut out, disconnected from our family abroad. This second-class connection with extended family is a loss and grief in and of itself. It is felt when we are not considered in major family decisions or not informed of major events because we are too far away. And though the distance placed between us and our families in Asia is not necessarily deliberate or malicious, the space between us can grow wide, as much as we may want to remain involved.

———— **REST STOP** ————

What losses have you experienced due to separation or disconnection from people and places in your homeland? What stories have you told yourself about these losses? Have you had a chance to acknowledge them and to grieve?

Loss through Trauma

When our parents (and grandparents, great-grandparents, and on) experience trauma, the effects can reach far through generations. Intergenerational trauma can be a powerful force, especially if it has not been processed or is outside of our awareness. Trauma, a felt sense that you are not safe, has the power to shape our behavior, perceptions, interpretations, and interactions. If your parents arrived in this country as refugees from a war-torn country, they react and respond to the world much differently than they would have if they arrived as graduate students beginning their education in a new country. Many conversations with clients and friends reveal that our parents' inability to show up well for us during childhood was due to the effects of post-traumatic stress or unresolved trauma from earlier parts of their lives. As we touched upon in chapter 3, it is not unusual for some of our parents to never have discussed or disclosed their trauma histories because it can be so overwhelming or terrifying. It is only after they have experienced spaces of safety and distance from these traumatic events that they may finally share with future generations about their painful memories. It is also possible that our parents will never share the most painful parts of their lives with us, and that is another source of grief that we might bear.

In the family context, intergenerational trauma can show up in many ways. At times, it appears as acts of abuse on future generations, as parents grapple with their own internal demons while also raising a family. Trauma can appear as a lack of emotional attunement or engagement, such as ignoring, dissociating, disappearing for hours or days at a time, or lack of empathy toward the emotions of others. Trauma can appear as explosive anger or involve emotional coercion as tools to shape the behaviors of others, such as physical or verbal abuse, threats of self-harm to get others to comply with requests, or threatening to expose personal secrets to force compliance from others. As with some of the other topics we've discussed, the realization of our parents' predecessors' challenges does not absolve them of responsibility; rather, it's important we highlight the impact of a person's pain on how they may deliberately or unintentionally inflict pain on others. One of the greatest losses we might experience as members of Asian diasporas is the loss of a parent we *wish* we could have had, if they had not experienced such trauma or painful experiences. There is loss in the relationship that *might have been* had they been spared from the life-altering events that impact many immigrant families.

Even to this day, my own mother lives in fear of her mother's explosive episodes. As a result, my mother was forced to learn absolute compliance and obedience as a way to protect herself from her mother's attacks. Even as a woman in her sixties, she defers to my grandmother, because any disagreement would result in the most violent verbal attacks on my mother's character, honor, and devotion as a daughter. I truly believe my grandmother suffered greatly at the hands of her own parents, who lived an agricultural existence and considered their children as a source of free labor. My grandmother's feelings of injustice and her rage about her own childhood were channeled toward my mother and her siblings as harsh, critical, and at times abusive parenting. In conversations with my mother, I can sense her deep sorrow about the many ways my grandmother could not be the mother she longed for and, even more painful still, about how she was robbed of a childhood.

REST STOP

How have the fingerprints of intergenerational trauma touched your life? Have you witnessed the effects of this trauma in your parents? In what ways? Are there losses that you have not been able to name due to the effects of trauma on your family?

Loss through Assimilation and Mimicry

As members of Asian diasporas, we are often placed in cultures and environments that are quite different from the cultures and customs of our homelands. Many of our countries of migration have complex and violent histories with individuals of Asian descent. Asian Americans have been vilified as perpetual foreigners while also touted as model minorities. Both stereotypes exert considerable impact on Asian immigrants from all waves of migration, as our phenotypic features do not allow us to pass within Western society. Code switching has become the norm, as our ability to adapt to different cultures and social expectations is the difference between being accepted or not. As a child, I became adept at code switching frequently between our Asian American community and my public-school setting. In white spaces, this allowed me to gain conditional acceptance and belonging, but it also resulted in a confused sense of identity. I struggled to reconcile the acceptable version of me that existed in white spaces with my Asian identity, which came through naturally, even though neither felt adequate to express the full person that I was becoming. My inability to articulate my sense of fractured identity kept me from understanding why I never felt whole for much of my life. This conflicted or confused identity reflects yet another layer of loss for us as children of diasporas.

In their book, *Racial Melancholia, Racial Dissociation*, professors David L. Eng and Shinhee Han explore the topic of racial melancholia, which they describe as a mourning without end for Asian Americans, a mourning for all of the parts of ourselves that cannot name the unknowable losses we experience as children of immigrants, as adoptees, as members of diasporas. The authors explore the cost of assimilation to and mimicry of white culture as a search for belonging, and the mourning that follows when we may realize that despite our best efforts, we are still never fully accepted. The heartbreaking part of this story is that in this mimicry of whiteness, we also sacrifice much of our own identity and histories in the process. What results is a dissociation and disconnection of the self in order to survive racism and xenophobia. In many immigrant households, parents chose not to speak in their native languages at home so as to ensure that their children learned fluent English—a skill that our immigrant parents may have lacked. In a bid to appear more Western, our families may have shed their cultural customs or rituals to make white neighbors, friends, or communities more comfortable. All of these cultural losses were the price of admission to a new home with ostensibly better opportunities and a safer existence. And yet, I believe that many of us are still mourning the loss of these intimate parts of ourselves that we had to hide in order to survive. So, we live in a space of perpetual mourning of our language, identity, and connectedness to our own people.

———— REST STOP ————

What are the losses you have experienced as a result of assimilation to white culture? How have these losses impacted you and your family? What assimilation losses would you like to reclaim at this point in your life?

NAMING THE LOSSES OF ASIAN DIASPORAS

In grief work, we are invited to trust the process of working through mourning, the understanding being that once we face our grief we will emerge, not cured, but matured, evolved, and eventually able to find freedom in the midst of it. Grief work doesn't involve an endpoint or deadline. Some say it's a lifelong weight we carry, and over time we get used to the burden, stronger beneath its bulk.

A number of the people I work with have tried to bypass grief, filling their time instead with busyness or distraction—only to realize that grief doubles down and demands to be addressed. Eventually, something will trigger this unacknowledged grief and the floodgates will open. With this in mind, the first step to understanding our grief is to uncover the sources of our loss, name them, and define them. When we name our grief, we start to localize our pain, we begin to understand it, and we may even invite it instead of trying to avoid it. That is when we can integrate the loss into our lives. This is why intergenerational trauma and grief, often unprocessed, have the potential to impact generations—because we carry a pain we may not be aware of and, in turn, inflict pain where we do not mean to. Grief that is acknowledged, processed, and held tenderly allows us to live with awareness of the pain but not displace it, not project it, and not hide from it either. In acknowledging our grief and holding it with compassion, we can dress the wound and give it a chance to heal.

In the following sections, we'll address some themes of loss that I have observed as a professional and as a member of an Asian diasporas. These themes are not exhaustive. They may be familiar to you—perhaps you've dealt with them all your life but had no words to define them; you may not have even realized you had these losses but felt them deeply, like a shadow following you through each season of life. As you uncover each, try to remember how, why, and when the losses impacted you. Can you trace back to the memories, images, or conversations in which you felt the loss? Can you notice how your body is responding to each named loss? Can you give yourself permission to feel the loss without trying to suppress or hold back? Can you allow your body to move through the emotion without trying to avoid it? Perhaps for you this may look like crawling into bed, crying, holding yourself or being held by a trusted person, going for a walk, watching a sad movie, or anything else that brings you comfort. Give yourself permission to do what is necessary to feel safe in your body in order to move through the excavated grief you might experience in this leg of the journey.

Loss of History and Lineage

The grief and pain associated with a lost history and disconnected lineage is one that even time cannot reconcile. For children of Asian diasporas, leaving our homeland means the trajectory of our cultural self and ethnic knowledge changes forever. We may become disconnected from customs, rituals, holidays, native faith traditions, ways of preparing food, healing practices, and so much more—and all of these disconnections reveal themselves over a lifetime. As we meet members of our community who have greater ties to our heritage, we may ache yet again for what we may have lost in our migration, whether it was by choice or not. And though our parents may have tried their best to instill the cultures, languages, and traditions of our homeland, there are certain experiences they could not replicate in our new countries.

In many ways, it feels as though I come from a people that I can trace only as far back as my grandparents. I don't even know the names of my great-grandparents, nor do I know about their stories. I will never long for Taiwan in quite the same way as my parents do or understand the meaning of being connected to ancestors. As an Asian American, my history is forever different from that of my Taiwanese cousins, and this fragmented history is something that I grieve as well. This sadness grows still as I realize that my children may be even further removed from our history and lineage. Part of our racial and ethnic identity development is impacted by our exposure to cultural pride and knowledge. It has taken me decades to arrive at a place of embracing my heritage and culture. Internalized racism caused me to run from my cultural heritage for much of my youth, believing my Asian-ness was somehow second class, something embarrassing. This is in part due to the loss I felt as a result of my displacement from my homeland.

When my grandfather passed on, I felt truly unanchored from my lineage for the first time in my life. He was my singular link to the people who came before me. He was the one adult of that generation who truly loved me, knew me, and showed me all of the beauty and honor of my heritage. He made me proud to be Taiwanese. It was through his lifeline that I felt belonging and recognition. When I was prohibited from seeing him one last time and unable to say goodbye, it left a gaping hole in my story and forever altered my sense of identity. In Asian diasporas, our loss is not just in the people we love or places that we miss; it is the loss of being grounded in a history of people who preceded you and from which you long to draw wisdom and strength.

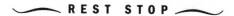

REST STOP

Do you feel connected to the history and culture of your people? What allows you to feel connected? What practices, rituals, or traditions help keep you linked to the history of your people? What about your disconnected history do you grieve? What do you wish you could access about your lineage? Where might you look for more connection?

Loss of Identity and Name

Our traditional Asian names represent our ties to our people who came before us. The strokes, sounds, and meanings of our names are often chosen with intention, meaning, and hope for the future. I was given the name Wang Tzu-Mei when I was born, because it was auspicious for my future. It was the name I carried until kindergarten, when I was teased for having a name that no one could pronounce. In an effort to make it easier for my teachers and classmates, my parents chose to replace my name with Jenny.

I was grateful at the time. I was relieved that I did not have to help others through the pronunciation of my name. I was glad that I'd no longer be teased every time the teacher took attendance. My American name protected me from the shame that I felt about my Asian-ness and allowed me a chance to "fit in." And yet, it also reinforced the narrative that my Asian-ness was not palatable enough for America. As young children, we could not have understood how stripping away our cultural names could impact our identity. We only knew that our Asian names were sources of pain, embarrassment, or shame. However, as adults, we may now realize that losing our names only worsened the internalized racism we experienced and only further fractured our identity.

───── R E S T   S T O P ─────

What are the origins of your name? What meaning or significance does it hold for you? Has your name evolved since you were born? If your name was changed, how has this impacted your Asian identity? What losses do you grieve about your identity and name?

Loss of Language and Stories

I recently asked my social media followers about the losses that they experience as members of Asian diasporas. One of the top responses was the loss of their native languages. Many expressed deep sadness over never being taught how to speak the languages of their ancestors or not having mastered them enough to communicate effectively with their parents and extended family. But it wasn't the inability to speak that was the primary loss, it was the struggle to connect with their parents and Asian family members that created the greatest sense of grief. Many expressed that they could not find the words to share their innermost feelings or discuss their needs, as language remained such a barrier between them and their parents. In effect, the lack of language silences us and keeps us from deeply knowing our history, our culture, and our parents, further widening the generational and cultural gaps between us. It also makes it much harder for us to communicate our emotions, needs, and points of view.

When language is stripped away, we also struggle to hear the stories that are necessary for us to feel connected to our people. Our parents may not be able to share their childhood experiences, memories, and struggles as the words may not translate well into English or other secondary languages. If we add on painful or traumatic memories that their childhoods may evoke, it only serves to create even more barriers to understanding and learning about our family stories. The grief of not being able to communicate with the people whom we long to understand the most remains an ongoing struggle for many children of Asian immigrants. For Asian adoptees, the lack of exposure to their native language may painfully remind them of the grief of being separated from their birth family and adopted in the first place. In many spaces, they may feel that their lack of knowledge of their Asian culture marginalizes them from their own Asian-ness. Language has the power to connect or divide people, and for those of us who struggle to speak our native tongues, it only highlights the disconnection that might exist between us and our ancestral people.

———— **REST STOP** ————

Do you speak the language of your ancestors? If so, what has this allowed you access to? If not, what has this locked you away from? What losses do you experience if you are unable to speak your native language fluently?

Loss of Belonging and Legacy

If a loss of history and lineage is a struggle to trace back to our roots, then a loss of belonging and legacy is the grief of not being able to ground ourselves as we look toward the future. As much as I have assimilated with my unaccented English and American education, I still feel the gaze of individuals who would rather make assumptions about me than actually speak to me and get to know me. The side-eye glances are no less penetrating than when I witnessed them directed at my parents almost twenty years ago. The undeniable impact of racism on Asian diasporas will leave us constantly doubting our abilities and questioning our belonging. Our tenuous acceptance may make us feel as though we must prove ourselves at every turn; we may feel that we're always on display at work, at school functions, and while navigating our neighborhoods. There is grief in being seen as "foreign, different, or other" at every table we are invited to. There is also grief in belonging just enough to be at the table, but not enough to be invited to share an opinion, make a suggestion, or assume leadership.

In this context of being seen as the perpetual foreigner, it is a struggle to envision a legacy that we are hoping to build for our future generations. The COVID-19 pandemic revealed a deep mistrust and fear of Asian people, as Asians were blamed for the outbreak of the virus in many Western countries, which unleashed unprovoked attacks on our people. As a mother of two young Asian American children, I fear for what they will face at school, at work, and in their neighborhoods one day. I worry that they will feel the same lack of belonging that many of us have felt our entire lives. I grieve over the loss of belonging for my children, who consider themselves American just as much as they are Asian. I mourn over the parts of themselves that they might learn to hate because our country values them conditionally—only if they are willing to fit the stereotype. It is hard to envision a legacy that will be left for our children to follow, as we are in the midst of fighting our own battles of belonging in the present day. I grieve the life my children could have experienced if they lived in a world in which they were part of the majority rather than the marginalized minority.

⟋ REST STOP ⟍

Do you have grief surrounding your sense of belonging or lack of belonging in your country? Are there parts of yourself you have had to hide away in order to gain that belonging? At what price? How do you grieve for the limitations and barriers that generations after you will need to endure?

The Gift of Grief

Perhaps it seems counterintuitive, but experiencing grief can help us see life through a new lens. It challenges our status quo and encourages us to reconsider the things we value. When we have suffered loss, we are forced to recognize that life is temporary, fleeting, and ever changing. In this fleeting nature, finding what grounds us becomes crucial. Grief also challenges us to intentionally consider how we want to live and what we want to change moving forward. While I am unable to provide how-to guidance for working through grief, as the path through grief is an intimate and unique one for each of us, I share with you one of my deepest spaces of grief with the hope that you can see how I have created space around my grief in order to see it with more clarity in the pain. In truth, even now this grief is with me and sometimes brings me to tears. And yet I continue to create space and tenderness around it in order to move through and keep myself from being consumed by it.

BEARING THE GRIEF

There are three needs of the griever: To find the words for the loss, to say the words aloud and to know that the words have been heard.

—VICTORIA ALEXANDER

Mourning rituals are a powerful and rich aspect of Asian cultural life. Many Asian ethnicities have exquisite and intentional practices surrounding how we are to grieve and mourn. In some cultures, we bring our loved ones forward in time with us in daily life by erecting small shrines within our homes to remember them. There are holidays at which we honor the dead by preparing their favorite foods and gathering items that we offer to our ancestors for their enjoyment. Death is an altering of the course of reality, but it is not an erasure of how that person remains in our lives or memories. We grieve openly and mourn with honor because we can fully identify and name the loss of a loved one. Their physical presence is gone from us, but they are not lost from our memories and daily lives. However, the grief of diasporic people takes on additional layers, as the sources of our grief cannot be isolated to a single object, person, or place. Our losses are made up of repetitive reminders of how we are cut off and disconnected from our culture and ancestors. The disconnection may have been so profound that we failed to realize they were losses at all.

It can feel as though the grief journey may threaten to destroy us when we approach it, but what we do know is that if grief is acknowledged, validated, and spoken, it is not destructive but instead gives freedom to the afflicted. When we learn how to grieve well, we are able to move more flexibly and gently through grief and joy, to move from the chaos caused by grief into deeper meaning. From heartache into purpose. From frantic longing into honored remembrance. As we carry our grief over seasons of life, we learn that grief may shift forms, contract or expand, and though the grief may never leave us, we strengthen our muscles for carrying its weight.

The most frustrating thing about grief is that there is no fixing it. Instead, we must create space for the grief to exist and to emerge when it needs to, and when it feels right, grieve with others who are capable of holding and seeing us in our pain. As much as our losses are individual, they are also collectively held as a community of people separated from their homelands. As you work through the following sections, your feelings of grief may actually increase as you allow yourself greater access to those painful parts. Doing this work will help you fear grief less and give you the opportunity to live in the grief without being consumed by it. I've provided these sections from my perspective, to show you how I worked through a particularly painful event, because when we grieve, we also develop deeper compassion for the pain and mourning of others. In the vulnerability of our grief, we are able to connect and access deeper, more honest parts of others as well. This is the reason we grieve, to allow us to connect in our grief with others and to strengthen those bonds around us in order to hold each other through the darkness.

Giving Grief a Name

In 2017, we tried to go back to Taiwan to see my grandparents. When my mother told my grandmother about our plan and that we were bringing her great-grandchildren back to meet them for the first time, it triggered an episode of intense anxiety and paranoia, after which my grandmother adamantly refused to allow us to return to Taiwan. She began to panic and worry about every possible negative outcome that might result from our trip. My grandmother's mental health status has always been a source of confusion for my family. I do not know her well enough, nor have I spent enough time with her to know what mental health conditions are impacting her, but something about her reasoning, judgment, and erratic behaviors has always felt concerning and alarming.

With three small children in tow, the trip would not be easy, but we were willing to take the more than twenty-four-hour journey to see our extended family, especially my grandfather. However, no matter how much convincing or reassurance my mother offered, my grandmother was unrelenting in her demands that we not visit. This rejection and blockage of our trip triggered so much anger and grief, and we eventually decided to visit Taiwan without my extended family's knowledge. We spent twelve days in Taipei on our own, and while we enjoyed our time together as a family, we were heartbroken that we could not see our grandfather during this trip, despite being less than an hour's train ride away from him. My mother feared that if my grandfather accidentally disclosed to my grandmother that we had visited, she would have another episode in which she would proceed to berate and terrorize my mother for months on end.

My grandmother demanded absolute obedience from my mother,

just as she always had since my mother was child. My mother's compliance and inability to break free from the cultural expectations of her generation broke my heart and felt like a profound loss—a loss of the mother I needed in the moment, who would fight for me and stand up for me, a mother who would stand up for herself in the face of her greatest challenge and threat, her own mother. And it was a loss of the opportunity for my grandfather to meet my children and my sister's child for the first time. And while I was prepared to fight my grandmother for the ability to visit, my mother was not, having been a victim of her mother's control for decades. So out of my respect and love for my own mother, I complied and relented.

This will be my greatest regret. My grandfather passed away eight months after our visit.

In my own journey of grief, I have come to realize that grief is not just sadness. Grief includes a whole host of emotions, such as disappointment, betrayal, anger, hopelessness, despair, regret, and more. This is the multilayered grief that exists for us, as children of diasporas. I still carry grief and anger over my mother's inability to fight for me and for her opportunity to see her father for the last time. Grief and anger over betrayal by my grandmother in robbing both of us of a chance to see my grandfather once more and robbing my children of the chance to meet their great-grandfather. Grief over the loss of my grandfather. Grief over being too far to travel back for his funeral. Grief over the lack of closure and the regret that my grandfather had no idea how much I longed to see him while he was alive. As painful as it has been, naming all of these forms of grief over this massive loss has given me clarity and helped me really understand why these losses are so painful to bear. This clarity has truly allowed me permission to feel and inhabit every ounce of these losses with nuance and granularity.

Naming our grief gives us strength to bear its weight. We now know what we carry. I can acknowledge the disappointment and frustration I feel toward my mother and also realize how difficult it must have been for her. I can hold space for my anger toward my grandmother while also understanding how her mental health and history caused so much havoc in her life. I can validate the ongoing pain I feel that my beloved grandfather is gone, having never met my children, and also recognize how important it is for them to know his story. I see all the layers of grief clearly, and it has provided some relief in the midst of the pain. It has also given me freedom to consider how I might think and live differently having suffered these losses.

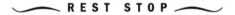

REST STOP

What lives in your space of grief? Is there something that you haven't yet given yourself permission to grieve? What are the multiple layers of grief that you may carry in your family, your migration, or in your identity as a member of an Asian diasporas?

Grief Spoken

In order to share this part of our story in this book, I knew I had to ask my mother for permission to include it, since it is as much her story as it is a part of mine. I avoided doing so for months, and it actually delayed the completion of this chapter. The thought of having to speak of my grief with my mother caused so much dread that it made me nauseous. I could not face her and the grief together; the idea of holding space for my grief and hers was too painful. I avoided this conversation because I knew it would unearth our shared grief over my grandfather once again, which had become a source of intense pain and regret for both of us. After a particularly convicting therapy session, I finally mustered up the courage to talk to my mother about my grandfather's passing— three years after he passed.

When my grandfather first left us, my mother called on a Saturday morning and said, "Ah Gong is gone." I remember I was in the middle of a run, and I stopped in my tracks, unable to breathe. The pain cut through me; it felt like a hot knife slicing through my stomach. As I walked through my front door, I saw my daughter and collapsed in tears. She ran over to me and asked, "Mommy, why are you crying?" I told her that my ah gong had just passed away. Since this is an affectionate term for "grandfather" in Taiwanese, it is the same name she calls my father, and she instantly made the connection—she understood that my loss felt to me as it would feel to her if she lost her own grandfather. Seeing my daughter also triggered more grief as I realized we had lost our chance for her to meet him. After that day, I packaged myself back up and just moved on with my life. We didn't pause to remember him. I never discussed with my mother how I felt. We just picked up and carried on much like we do, as immigrants and members of an Asian diasporas. We just pushed through.

It wasn't until I began writing this book that I realized I would need to confront this grief at some point, that I would need to breathe life into this part of my story in order to share this chapter with you. I realized that without speaking my grief out loud and bringing it into existence with the one person who understood the depth of my pain, I could not move forward and heal. A few nights ago (I wasn't lying when I said I had avoided this conversation until now), I called my mother over video. I said to her, "I am writing a chapter on grief, and I just cannot move on. I miss Ah Gong so much." And then I burst into tears. My mother then proceeded to cry with me as she expressed how much she also missed her own father. We shared about our anger, our pain, our regrets, and our struggles as we had each waded through the past three years of our grief alone. And while the grief lingers still, speaking about my grief with the one person who would understand has allowed me to breathe a bit easier. It opened the door for us to bring up my grandfather in conversation more easily.

Speaking about our grief allows us to keep our lost ones, lost parts, and lost seasons with us. It breaks down the walls of compartmentalization and avoidance and allows us to access the full richness of having loved, experienced, and lived fully. Speaking about our grief also provides us with connection to others. It is a balm that temporarily soothes those aching parts of ourselves and reminds us that we are not alone.

REST STOP

What parts of your grief may need to be spoken about and given space to exist outside of yourself? How might you create space to acknowledge your grief? Consider conversations like the one I had with my mother or through art, dance, movement, song, writing, therapy, etc. How can you speak about or express your grief so that you can truly feel and allow it to move through you?

Grief Inhabited, Grief Understood

As much as I may long to fix how my story ended with my grandfather, I cannot change the past or the decisions that were made. I cannot change my grandmother's struggle with mental health or the dynamics that she and my mother have had for six decades. All I can do is take this experience of grief and allow myself to understand the losses, not fear them as much, and see what my grief may reveal to me about my own life. I always share with clients that grief is the other side of the coin of love. It is only with deep love that we are even capable of experiencing such deep grief. On the days when the grief does not feel as hard, I look at the other side of the coin. What lives in that space of things that I might have lost and now would like to somehow reclaim and reintegrate into myself? I step fully into my grief in order to see what existed before the loss that I can bring more intentionally into my life.

As my mother shared about her painful relationship with her own mother throughout her childhood, I asked, "Then how did you know how to raise us? When you were treated so poorly by your own mother, how did you learn how to love your own children with so much warmth and compassion?" She said, "Because I knew that your grandfather was a part of me too. He taught me that." My mother fully recognized that she could have ended up like her own mother if she allowed all of her trauma, pain, and abuse to consume her. She could have lashed out at my sister and me. She could have displaced the legacy burdens of her mother and grandmother onto us, thereby perpetuating the cycles of harm and pain throughout future generations. But she didn't. She broke the cycle in one generation. She stepped into her grief over the childhood she never had, the mother she struggled to love, and the loss of a father who taught her how to love, and stepped out on the other side knowing that she had to live differently in order to give my sister and me a different trajectory in life. This is how she inhabited her grief and moved through to the other side of it.

When we understand our grief, we begin to see life differently. We start to understand how our grief reveals the parts of ourselves and our lives that are true and are most important. We develop a self-knowing that no one is able to take away. We see through the noise of life and understand what is truly valuable and should be cherished. As I have slowly excavated my own multilayered grief surrounding my Asian identity, I have come to see with clarity the stories that I have been hiding for my entire life in order to keep myself safe. I have come to see that I no longer need those stories as protection. I no longer need to fit any stereotype in order to be accepted, because I am now capable of providing myself with the things I lacked as a young child of immigrants. And though I still feel sadness for all that I lost in my migration, I can also see all that I have gained in the journey too and have developed the ability to hold space for both. Going forward, I will try my best to offer what I have learned through my grief to my children as we build together with them a history, a community, and a lineage that I always longed for. My grief and pain have given way to a fire to help my children know their history, culture, lineage, and people. And my intentional reclaiming of these parts for myself has given my children access to their ancestry and heritage as well.

⁓ REST STOP ⁓

Please give yourself space and time to experience your grief before asking yourself these questions. *After mourning and feeling your grief, what has been revealed to you? What clarity does your grief offer you about what you love, cherish, and value in this life? How might you begin to offer yourself what you need in your spaces of grief, as a member of an Asian diasporas? What steps can you take to move toward those needs? For some people, this has looked like reclaiming their Asian names, taking language classes, seeing their parents more often to hear stories, reading books with their children about their history and lineage, writing about their lived experiences, and/or sharing with friends about their experiences of racism.*

*   *   *

As we close this chapter, I hope you have had moments to pause and to tune into your grief, as a child of immigrants, as a member of a diasporas. Know that your grief, though painful, will not destroy you if you allow yourself permission to experience it. You are capable of withstanding the pain of holding your grief, and I would encourage you to find people who are able to hold you as you create space for your grief. And though I cannot promise what specifically will be waiting for you on the other side of your mourning, I can tell you that there is richness and freedom there— richness in being able to see and live life on your own terms, based on what is most important to you, and freedom in being able to breathe and live well in the midst of the grief that remains. Your grief exists to show you that which you love most. Give yourself the opportunity to move through your grief to find the most beautiful parts of yourself, your life, and your culture that you might reclaim along this journey.

CHAPTER 10

Permission to Come Home

Home is not where you were born; home is where all your attempts to escape cease.

—OMAR TAHER

I titled this book *Permission to Come Home* long before I was certain of its contents. I knew for sure that I wanted to end in this space of homecoming and return, one in which we have evolved, matured, and grown from the inner child most of us still carry within us. I spent many of my years running away from the spaces that caused me great pain and yet also longed intensely to find peace, constantly feeling a push and pull in so many different parts of my life—with my parents, within my culture, within my Asian American–ness—only to discover that in order to find freedom, peace, and my true self, I needed to take the difficult journey through the hurt, disappointment, and resentment to build a space I could recognize as home.

Up until this point, our journey has been terrestrial. We have intentionally walked off the beaten path to glimpse what our lives might look like outside of the rules, frameworks, and expectations we have been bound by. My hope is that you have allowed yourself to sink deep into the previous chapters to intentionally challenge and question how you think about and show up in your world. I hope you see that perhaps you have been playing out stories that have actually been keeping you from finding your home and how these stories tend to tell you lies: lies about your worth, lies about who you must be in order to belong, lies about what really makes you valuable, and lies about how you must betray yourself in order to be liked and accepted. With new awareness of these untruths, I hope you now can allow yourself to grieve and mourn the parts of you that need shedding in order for you to find your way home. Home may look different to us as members of Asian diasporas than we imagined, hoped for, or thought it to be. And yet, this does not diminish our story, but in fact makes our homecoming even more meaningful.

In the previous chapters, you have been hard at work breaking down the barriers that have been keeping you stuck. You've been rethinking the way you want to move forward. You have tripped and fallen over your old roadblocks, and yet you courageously continue. The road ends here. Now, we must take to the waters, to the unexplored spaces that have no clearly marked routes but instead invite you to chart your own course. As Asian diasporas, we left our homes by crossing oceans, and so the return to our proverbial home means entering the waters once again to find the space where we can exist with authenticity, belonging, and peace. In starting this part of the journey, you might notice a stir of fear and anxiety about the unknown. It can be disquieting to think about the person you could become should you decide to step beyond your comfort zone. You may have fears: What if you try and others don't approve? What if you don't succeed at achieving the life you want to build? Maybe it's easier, then, to not try at all. But what if? What if you finally gave yourself permission to live outside of all that used to keep you small, stuck, and trapped?

If you listen closely, there might also be a quieter part of you that feels a thrill and excitement over the potential and possibilities that await. At sea, there are no walls to block you or roads you must stick to. You are free. You claim freedom when you realize that so many of us are trapped by the repeated stories we tell ourselves about who we are and what is possible in this life. You find freedom when you see that society has created rules steeped in hierarchy, patriarchy, misogyny, homophobia, transphobia, xenophobia, classism, ableism, racism, and other -ias and -isms in order to keep us tame. When you see the fortresses that have been erected around you your entire life, you gain the clarity you need to break free, explore on your own terms, and decide how you want to live. It means cherishing the parts of ourselves and cultures that nourish our identities and leaving behind the parts that no longer serve. When we continue our journey by sea, we learn the art of reading our own compass perhaps for the first time in our lives.

As we begin the last leg of our journey together, I invite you to give yourself permission to finally come home. This may be a complicated idea for those of us who do not have a specific place we call home. Home, instead, could be a person, or feeling, or a mentally constructed space. As much as it pains me to admit, Taiwan is not my home. Despite my pride for my culture and heritage, it is not my home. It is a place I long for and grieve over in my heart, but it is not a home that knows me with intimacy. I've spent so much of my life in the United Sates, but I am not yet certain I can call it my home either. It neither knows me nor accepts me as I am. What has become apparent to me is that home is a space that we must cultivate ourselves, deliberately and intentionally. It is a space we must co-create with those we love and bring into existence wherever we are.

——— R E S T   S T O P ———

What is your idea of home? Where does it exist for you? How does being at home make you feel in your body and mind? Who is there waiting for you when you return home?

DEFINING YOUR HOME

I can recognize moments of being at home because I feel it in my body. I feel my muscles relax, my breathing slows and paces naturally, my mind feels at ease, and I do not need to remain alert in case there is danger. It makes sense that home is much more about a physical and psychological state of being than it is a physical location or country. James Baldwin wrote, "Perhaps home is not a place, but simply an irrevocable condition." Is it possible that home is simply a space from which we cannot be turned away, turned out, or denied? In the midst of all the fleetingness and uncertainty in this life, home is the one place that offers a bit more permanence or stability; it is a space we can return to again and again in spite of feeling or being shut out elsewhere.

I recently asked my social media community what home looks like for them, and several of the responses listed specific people, like mothers, partners, or their own children. There's a reason a feeling of home can be located within relationships. Theories around child development suggest our primary caregivers or first attachment figures often make up our "secure base," a psychological and physical space in which we are able to return after we venture out to explore our world. When my daughter was thirteen months old, we would visit the local neighborhood library for story time and playtime. At first, she would hesitate to leave my side, but as the teacher introduced musical instruments—tambourines, shakers, and cymbals—she was naturally drawn toward these instruments and wandered away from me. But every once in a while, I would observe her realize the distance between us and crawl back with an instrument in hand to show me and explore together.

I realize not all of us had a chance to develop this psychological secure base. In cases of neglect, abuse, or disconnection, we may have struggled to develop a secure place with our primary caregivers. Instead, it is possible that our parents in their own struggles with trauma, mental health, or poverty and hardship could not offer themselves as the safe and secure place to which we could return when we felt scared and alone. My work with clients reveals many similar stories, in which clients recall being largely ignored by their parents or left alone for much of their childhood. And as a result, they had to develop their own protective mechanisms to ward off their fears of abandonment or being unlovable. Some develop impenetrable walls of independence and try to prove to themselves and everyone else that they can survive as an island. They struggle to connect intimately with others out of fear that if they become attached to someone, that person will eventually leave and they would be devastated. Others develop intense anxiety and panic when their loved ones are not physically near them. They struggle with being alone or engaging in life independently because they feel incapable of handling the anxiety of being alone. Notice how all of these behaviors are born out of our childhood needs to survive a space that feels unsafe, unloving, or scary. This is not a personal flaw; this is our minds and bodies needing to survive at all costs with the cards we are dealt.

In identity work, part of the transformation happens when we begin crafting and developing our own secure base. As we enter adulthood, if we have felt safe, loved, and cherished, we begin to internalize a secure base within ourselves. We begin to shape and craft an identity that feels worthy, valuable, loved, and connected with others. Our primary caregivers, by showing us love, affection, and safety, allow us to create an internal self-concept that is able to love, provide safety, and cherish ourselves. In the best-case scenario, we become our own secure base that is interconnected with those we love. But if we lack these positive reinforcements from our primary caregivers, we begin to internalize false messages about who we are. We might believe that we are flawed, broken, unlovable, and incompetent and deserve to be alone. As a result, we may spend our lives searching for a secure base in others but be unable to recognize what a secure base looks like. We might date or marry partners who reinforce our "not good enough" narratives instead of offering us the love and safety that we so desperately seek. We may feel panicked if we are without a companion or partner, because being alone activates our abandonment fears and triggers the story that we are not worthy of love. This is why we must learn how to identify what home may look like for each of us, what our secure base provides us, and how to find these spaces or cultivate them with intention.

Throughout this chapter, I have homed in on the four elements that create a secure base: safety, belonging, authenticity, and compassion. These cardinal directions help to identify whether a space feels like home or not. In my life, some spaces meet only two or three out of the four conditions, but kindred sacred spaces meet all four of my conditions for home. When a space reflects all four of these conditions, I feel at home, and the less it reflects these conditions, the less it feels like home. You can use these tools to help you identify what a space needs to have for you to feel at home.

Not all spaces will fulfill all four cardinal points. In fact, some may not reflect any of these conditions at all, but this doesn't mean that we avoid these spaces altogether. Instead, it means our goals or hopes for entering what could be an unsafe space must outweigh the cost of lacking safety, belonging, authenticity, and compassion. I offer a circumstance from my own life: As a trainee in graduate school, I often felt that I needed to hide. I had to code switch in order to be considered professional enough to earn my degree. I rarely felt safe as I was under the evaluation and gaze of white supervisors who tried their best to shape me into what they thought a psychologist should look, think, and behave like. I was not encouraged to live authentically but actually to conform to the values and standards of Western psychology. While I felt belonging within my cohort, I did not always experience a sense of belonging within the predominantly white graduate training program. And though I experienced compassion from specific supervisors or mentors, it often felt conditional, provided that I followed the rules and kept my head down. However, I entered that space, a place I could not call home, with the greater goal of being able to earn my degree and licensure and one day serve and represent our community. The future goal outweighed the cost of having to navigate a space that often did not feel like home.

As you read, I encourage you to consider what your personal conditions are for feeling at home. Perhaps there is some overlap with the four conditions I share here, or you have unique requirements that help you feel at home. What might they be? How do these conditions make you feel when they are present?

Safety

Safety is a nonnegotiable first condition for a space to feel like home, because home is the space in which we can retreat from outside threats. With safety, we are able to be open-minded, creative, and engaged, and we can explore without fear. It is the space in which we can ask questions without being called stupid; we can make suggestions and have them be genuinely considered. It is the space in which we believe that we will not be subject to threat or attack. Safety forms the basis of connection to others. Without safety, home cannot exist.

I generally feel safe in most areas of my life: work, marriage, friendships, parents, siblings, children. However, when I enter predominantly white spaces, my sense of safety drops to varying degrees based on my familiarity with that space. I become watchful and careful. I scan my environment and people's reactions, and I consider how I may be represented toward them. This vigilance, awareness, and scanning is extremely exhausting. Home is a place that does not deplete, but rather replenishes, and moving toward spaces of greater safety or finding enclaves in which we experience safety to balance spaces that lack safety may become important self-care.

─── **REST STOP** ───

Give yourself a moment to consider all the spaces you inhabit. How much safety exists in each of those spaces? As the level of safety diminishes, how does this impact your perceptions of whether this feels closer to or further away from an idea of home? How might you increase your sense of safety in certain spaces?

Belonging

When we feel as though we belong, it can offer a sense of comfort and familiarity. The sense of being accepted into a group has been an important part of primal human experience for centuries. A sense of belonging has allowed us to survive many centuries on this planet. So, belonging is another condition that must be met in order for me to feel at home within a space. Belonging often means that there are threads of connection between people; it means we can deepen relationships, because there is a basic level of belonging through group membership.

However, belonging has its limits in terms of how closely we can reach a space of home. We can belong to a group but also feel dreadfully alone. We can be considered a part of a team and feel as though we are invisible and silenced. Simply by being an employee of a company, we could say that we belong to that group, and yet we can also feel as though we are not considered a valuable contributor to the organization. Our needs, opinions, and wants are often not actually seen or heard. While belonging can bring us one step closer to a sense of home, we need more than just safety and belonging to call a place home.

—— R E S T S T O P ——

Which spaces offer you a sense of belonging? Does the sense of belonging expand beyond being a member of a group? Do these group members see you, know you, and value you?

Authenticity

As we move toward a deeper sense of home, authenticity is the next condition that must exist. So much of my Asian American, female, heteronormative experience has been about shape-shifting and people-pleasing. When I am able to be authentic in a space, I can feel it instantly. There are no pretenses. I am able to make mistakes without punishment or shame. I can fail and realize that the failure is part of my growth. And I am invited to be vulnerable and show my weakest parts without fear that I will be rejected or found unworthy. Authenticity moves us closer to home because now we are more than just safe or part of a group; we are actually able to be our full, unfiltered selves. What a gift it is to find spaces like this. When we can be authentic, we are truly one step closer to home.

—— R E S T   S T O P ——

What spaces can you live in authentically, without hiding or masking? How does your body feel in these spaces? Who is there in this space? Does it feel closer to what home might feel like?

Compassion

This final condition is one of the most elusive and rare to find in our search for home. But compassion, the experience of being held and seen, may be one of the most intimate and sacred signposts that point us toward home. We can have safety, belonging, and authenticity, but the experience of being received and held with compassion and care is almost magical. So many factors make it difficult for us to feel truly held in someone's focused attention and compassionate presence. Many of us are so distracted and busy that making time to slow down enough to hold another in our compassionate attention is truly difficult. We also struggle to hold someone in compassion without the urge to fix, minimize, or reduce their suffering or struggle. Few of us have learned the art of listening to hold another in compassion versus listening to fix. In my experience, a space that allows us to share vulnerably and to be held in another's gaze, presence, and attention feels the closest to home that I think many of us will ever come.

Personally, one of the losses I still grieve is how my parents have offered ample safety, belonging, and space for authenticity but still struggle to hold me in compassion. Sometimes I wonder if it is the generational and cultural gaps that make it difficult for them to truly see me and hold me. They love me so dearly that I know they are trying their best to hold me in the ways that they can, but their own worries and anxieties often get in the way. Their own frameworks for living make it difficult for them to truly hold me in a space of attunement. When I shared with them my opportunity to write this book, they initially seemed neither excited nor proud. They did what many immigrant parents of a certain age did: worry. Would I be able to write it? Would I get ripped off in the process? Their mistrust of Western systems is still a pervasive part of their frameworks. I worked through this in therapy, fully recognizing that they were operating out of their own mindsets and perspectives of safety, scarcity, and anxious concern, but feeling heartbroken that my parents were unable to move into a space of realizing what I needed most from them was a shared acknowledgment and celebration of this accomplishment. And while I do not blame them for not being able to enter that celebratory space with me at first, I had to grieve the loss of not being fully held by them after all these years. Being seen and truly held can be a difficult space to find, but when you do, you are that much closer to home.

REST STOP

Where are the spaces in which you feel most seen and heard? What does it feel like when you are held in someone's focused compassion? How does your body feel when you are seen and held in someone's compassionate attention? Does this feeling feel closer to home?

THE WAY HOME IS THROUGH

When my daughter was born, she was given a book called *We're Going on a Bear Hunt*. It's a repetitive book in the way children's books are, in which a group of children are on a bear hunt and encounter a snowstorm, a thick swamp, tall grass, and all different kinds of natural conditions along their journey to catch a bear. There's a line that recurs: "We can't go over it. We can't go under it. We have to go through it." It's uncanny how accurately this simple book frames our experience of navigating life and our search for home. If we go over it or under it and bypass the journey through the hardship, pain, struggle, and sorrow, we just might keep ourselves from finding our space of peace within ourselves, our families, and our cultures.

I believe that I am now at the point of continual arrival and homecoming. In the past, the painful memories and hurtful dynamics kept me from seeing that there was a way through, but I now know and can see when I am headed in the wrong direction or am headed toward what feels like home. When I am headed the wrong way, when I lack safety, belonging, authenticity, or compassion, I believe I am valuable enough to course correct, say no, change my mind, or fight back in order to claim my right to journey home.

As I look over my life, I have had to confront four spaces in order to return home. This process has been challenging; it has involved verbalizing the hard stuff, the difficult stuff. It's involved questioning my culture and being told it was disrespectful and dishonoring to my elders. It took fighting all my "not good enough" stories to believe that I could fight against structures that kept me small and silent. But in approaching, inviting in, and embracing these four painful spaces in my life, which housed the majority of my trauma and pain, I have finally found freedom and a semblance of home within myself, the relationships I value the most, and the spaces I inhabit.

I offer these examples to encourage you to consider the spaces that you may need to wade through in order to return home, the spaces that have caused you pain and anguish and that you may have trouble facing because of how hurtful they have been. If this feels unsafe to do on your own, perhaps entering this phase of your journey with a trusted friend, sibling, or even a professional mental health clinician can help support you in understanding the spaces that keep you from finding your way home.

Finding Home through Systems and Structures

One of the most impactful paths I have had to take in my journey home has been traversing the murky waters of violent systems that have caused harm to my identity and self-concept. During the COVID-19 pandemic, Asians across the world watched in horror as they witnessed repeated attacks on our elderly, women, and even children. These instances triggered memories and experiences of our own racial trauma from the past that many of us may have suppressed or minimized over the years. In a country that has largely ignored and minimized—almost to the point of invisibility—the racial trauma of Asian Americans, we have had to confront the ways in which racism, xenophobia, and violence have impacted our psychological lives and identities.

There's no way we could have been prepared for the harmful interactions that we experienced in our childhoods or adult lives. While we felt the effects of racism, we were largely advised to ignore them, or worse yet, we were blamed for the discrimination we experienced. You might have been told, "This is happening because you weren't good enough. You didn't try hard enough. If you had done better, this may not have happened." Instead of naming the harmful and toxic effects of surviving whiteness, patriarchy, misogyny, ableism, transphobia, homophobia, and more, these structures were unnamed and unchallenged, and so instead, we blamed ourselves. We believed that perhaps we were mistreated because we were flawed, not good enough, or had done something wrong. This self-blame for external violent systems and structures insistent on maintaining the status quo is how we have come to internalize the self-hatred that many of us may carry within ourselves. This self-hatred that has kept us from finding our way home.

On the journey home, I have given myself permission to name these systemic forces. As I have come to see with clarity the toxic structures in place in my life, I realize my default mode does not always have to be to bend, mold, and defer, but instead I have the freedom to choose when I will fight, self-advocate, question injustice, and decide that spaces are too toxic to continue to remain in. It has meant leaving spaces that do not honor my dignity, ethics, and values. It has involved calling out injustice versus making myself believe that a personal flaw brought this harm upon myself. When I name the harm that is directed at me, I can shield and protect against it without allowing it to damage my sense of self. And in this self-created protection, I created a greater sense of home in spite of the structures I must live in.

───── **REST STOP** ─────

What systems and structures have kept you from finding value and worth within yourself? What self-hatred or self-blame has been created for you by these systems? Can you give yourself permission to name these harmful systems and realize how they may have created harmful narratives about yourself?

Finding Home through Culture

For Asian diasporas, cultural identity may have been a source of complexity and confusion. Being raised in a culture outside of our parents' cultures and having to navigate Western cultures largely unguided, it may seem impossible to find a home in such a conflicted space. A number of my clients express a feeling of being torn or having to choose between two or more cultures. This tension sometimes holds us hostage, as we feel like we have to compromise, suppress, or hold back in order to honor the expectations of each culture, or we feel ourselves pulled within the obligations and duties that our culture seems to place on us.

In coming home to my cultural identity, I have come to understand that perhaps the push/pull isn't to my detriment but adds optionality to my life. Instead of being completely bound to one framework or way of living out my culture, I am able to pick and choose cultural elements from my multicultural background to create a life that I want to live. I can simultaneously relish my sense of interconnectedness within my Asian cultural values while also communicating and lovingly setting boundaries to protect myself and my energy. I can pass along my cultural customs and practices to my children while also not transmitting intergenerational trauma onto them. I can learn how to discuss my mental health openly and dispel the shame around vulnerability while also honoring my family and culture by living a healthy, meaningful, and fulfilling life. As bicultural or multicultural individuals, perhaps we can view this multifaceted cultural heritage as a gift that gives us more freedom to choose.

In the journey back home to my culture, I have come to see all the benefits and richness of my cultural identity as well as all the parts that keep me from finding home. Should cultural elements put me in a position of having to compromise my felt sense of safety, belonging, authenticity, or compassion, I now am aware enough to question whether this cultural value is something I must adhere to or if there is an alternative way to engage so that I do not need to compromise my sense of home within my culture. One primary space I am learning to release from in my cultural upbringing is the culture of shame. I will no longer allow myself to move into a place of self-imposed or externally imposed shame. I have come to see that my weaknesses inform my identity and give me powerful knowledge about how to live my life. Shame is antithetical to my sense of home—my safety, belonging, authenticity, and compassion—and I refuse to surround myself with people or spaces that use shame as a motivator or source of coercion. Finding our way home through our culture means seeing that culture is simply a lens through which to see and engage our world, and we, as members of Asian diasporas, are fortunate that we can access multiple lenses at once.

—— REST STOP ——

What aspects of your cultural identity do you cherish and value the most? What cultural elements make you feel at home and give you a place of safety, belonging, authenticity, and compassion? What parts of your culture lead you further away from home?

Finding Home through Relationships

When people hurt you repeatedly, it can be easy to move to a space of anger, blame, and self-protection to ward off future pain. But this space isn't one of healing. It only pushes down the emotion temporarily until another trigger invariably sets off another emotional event. As I shared in chapter 2, my father has repeatedly hurt me—not physically, not in the abusive sense, but rather, he lacked the warmth and encouragement I desired from him. In response, I lashed out, stonewalled, distanced, and tried to protect myself from the constant sense of criticism and disappointment that I felt from him. In this state of protectiveness, I could not let go, forgive, or move past these painful encounters. Instead, I stewed and waited until the next infraction to pounce back.

I know very little about my father's childhood aside from bits and pieces of memories or stories that he chooses to share. My understanding is that his family was cold, strict, and highly critical. I have no knowledge of direct trauma, but there were likely painful events that resulted in the person he is today. One of the most painful parts of our relationship is that he may never be the engaged, warm, and optimistic father many of my friends may have had growing up. I have come to terms with this, although it is still awkward when we hug and when I tell him I love him, but I do it anyway. It pains me that more often than not his words hurt me more than uplift me, and that my interactions with him cause me anxiety and panic rather than comfort and safety. These are remnants of his own upbringing and life experiences that I carry as a legacy burden as his daughter. So, I mourn the loss of the lighthearted, emotionally attuned, and compassionate father figure that I wish I had. I hold this in tension with the father that he is and the love that he shows in the ways he knows how. As I have come to mourn this loss of what I desired from him, this mourning has given me freedom to accept and embrace the father that he is capable of being and letting that be enough in the midst of my loss.

There may be people who, for your own mental health and

self-protection, you cannot keep in your life, and in that case, taking steps to distance yourself is vital to your mental health. For those who you are able to stay connected with, finding your way home through these relationships means accessing and acknowledging the pain first. When you get in touch with your own pain and hurt, it increases your capacity to see the pain and hurt of others—even in a person who has hurt you. As I have come to see my father as much more than a two-dimensional, stereotypical stoic Asian father, I feel less trapped by our painful past. I am able to see my old dynamics with him and step back enough to sometimes show up differently with him. And when I relate to him from a more grounded, confident, and compassionate space, he has actually learned to shift into this more regulated place as well. This doesn't entirely free us of conflict, but when he does wound me, I can name, explain, and understand it well enough that it no longer consumes me or makes me question my worth. As I have learned how to regulate myself in my interactions with my father, he has also learned how to co-regulate with me, and in that we have found a space in which we can finally exist as ourselves and find a piece of home with each other.

⟋⟍ REST STOP ⟋⟍

Are there relationships in your life you struggle to find a common ground or place of home in? What have your patterns been in these relationships? Have you allowed yourself to truly acknowledge, hold, and process your pain within these relationships? If not, why not? How can you create safety and protection around yourself so that you can allow access to these painful relationships? What does accessing the pain reveal to you?

Finding Home through the Self

The final piece of my journey home is the path through myself, through which I've seen how all the previous layers of systems and structures, culture, and personal relationships have contributed to how I view myself and my place in the world. Without breaking down how all of these influences contributed to my identity and self-concept, I never would have arrived at a season of my life in which I feel at home in my own mind, body, and skin. When we are able to visualize the frameworks restricting us, we are then able to access the freedom to choose something different.

On the other side of the journey through these painful layers is what I believe could be your home: Home in a self that is more whole and integrated with the freedom to acknowledge all your hurtful experiences, without the fear that you will be destroyed by them. Home in relationships where you remain a part of the equation, able to vocalize your needs, wants, and frustrations without the risk of abandonment or being cut off. Home within your culture for all those parts that you choose to keep and all the parts that you choose to leave behind without the fear of bringing shame or disrespect to your family or community. Home even within the harsh and harmful structures that you may face every day in public, at work, or even within your families without fear that these structures will diminish your value or dignity. Home in yourself, when you witness the injustice in these structures and can, perhaps, combat them and build a world that is more equitable and just for future generations.

Finding our way home means learning new stories about who we are, what we are capable of, the people that matter to us, and where we are headed. By living in these new stories, we unlock the unimaginable potential for ourselves to build a life we get to live. We can envision an expansiveness in developing relationships that we care about, in building a life of purpose and meaning, and in becoming a person we can't quite imagine yet today. As members of Asian diasporas, when we find our home within ourselves, we realize that we can be powerful without needing to oppress or dominate, we can experience deep emotion without feeling destroyed by it, we can honor ourselves while honoring others, we can locate ourselves in multiple cultures and hold space for our losses as well, and we can be authentic in who we are while not shaming or guilting ourselves for never being enough.

——— R E S T   S T O P ———

What would it feel like for you to find a home within yourself? What types of new stories might you need to tell yourself in order to feel closer to your home? How might you challenge the stories that rob you of safety, belonging, authenticity, and compassion in your life?

CHARTING NEW WATERS

In our final exercise, I encourage you to consider the four spaces introduced in this chapter: systems and structures, culture, relationships, and the self. Explore the narratives that exist within each space about who you are allowed to be, the rules that exist in each, and whether or not you want to continue abiding by these frameworks. Give yourself permission to question and challenge the stories that no longer serve you and be open to the potential of finding and writing new stories for yourself.

Moving through Systems and Structures:

Current storylines and narratives: What rules, obligations, expectations, or limitations exist in the systems and structures that impact your life? For example, patriarchy, misogyny, racism, ableism, transphobia, homophobia, classism, and so on.

Challenging frameworks: How do you feel about these structures in your life? How do these structures play out in your life, and are they serving you? How might you challenge these structures and counter-argue the messages they impart on you and your place in this world?

Building anew: What new stories or narratives could you consider that might bring you more safety, belonging, authenticity, and compassion?

Moving through Your Culture(s):

Current storylines and narratives: What are the aspects of your culture that feel most difficult for you to navigate? Why are they difficult for you?

Challenging frameworks: Do you believe that adhering to these cultural elements is serving you and helping you build the life that you want? What are the barriers that are keeping you from building that life?

Building anew: What might you need to let go of in your culture in order to build your desired life? What would you like to keep from your culture moving forward? How can you honor your culture yet give yourself permission to create an identity that feels like home?

Moving through Your Relationships:

Current storylines and narratives: Which relationships feel or felt the hardest for you in your life? What storylines have you developed over time to explain these difficult relationships and how you show up in them?

Challenging frameworks: Are these relationship dynamics serving you? Are they improving these relationships, or are they keeping you stuck in cycles of hurt, anger, and pain? What might you be avoiding in these relationships that is making it difficult to move forward?

Building anew: What might you need to acknowledge, name, and access in order to tend to the hurt parts of yourself within these relationships? How might you show up differently in these relationships? How can you sidestep the patterns and engage from a more grounded, regulated space?

Moving through Yourself:

Current storylines and narratives: What stories have you been telling yourself over time? How did these stories develop?

Challenging frameworks: What evidence exists for the truth of these stories now? How much of these stories were reflections of the hurt, pain, or baggage of others that were projected onto you?

Building anew: What new stories might you tell yourself about who you are and the value you have in this world? When you step outside of the stories of others, what remains in that space? What harsh, critical stories might you need to release in order to find home within yourself?

*   *   *

As we close this chapter and come to the end of our journey together, I hope you were able to catch glimpses of what home might look like for you. It may not be a specific place, person, or even idea. Home may be a feeling, an experience, or a condition of being. Finding our way home is not easy when so many influences in our lives have tried to obscure the path. And yet, we persist. We place trust in the knowledge that there is more truth and more meaning out there to be found. In your search for home, perhaps you will discover that the way there is through yourself, that as you travel inward to discover the darkness that has touched your life, you also will find the light that exists beside it. Your journey reveals the spaces in your life that offer safety, belonging, authenticity, and compassion, and now you can begin to recognize them as places you can call home. You can find the way back to your culture by building a new home within it, one that does not strip away your uniqueness but enhances the many parts of yourself that this world desperately needs. You find your way home not so that you can settle and hide there for the rest of your life, but so that you know the way back to a space that offers comfort, rest, and affirmation of your unshakable value and worth—an irrevocable worthiness, in spite of what the world may tell you, so that you can fully embark on the expansive and boundless adventure that is your life.

Final Thoughts

Thank you for taking this journey with me. In traveling together, the road felt less burdensome, and the stumbling blocks felt easier to overcome, because I was writing for you, for me, and for my kids, Evie and Theo, who will one day be young Asian American adults navigating the very complexities you and I are struggling through. I wrote this book as a way to document my pilgrimage and those of my clients, as we have taken the difficult, unmarked path home. I did not anticipate the emotional and psychological toll that writing this book would take, as I could not write from my head but instead had to write from the most vulnerable and tender spaces within myself. There were many nights when I felt exhausted from having to uncover, name, and share the painful stories within my life in order to offer tangible examples and real-life experiences that you might relate to, as children of Asian diasporas. So, I want you to know that if this work feels exhausting, triggering, and overwhelming, please don't think that you are somehow doing this work in the wrong way. Instead, understand these signs as cues indicating a need for additional self-care and support from family, friends, or a trained mental health professional to help carry the weight of your work. It is precisely because this work is so tiresome and painful that many of us try to avoid it.

Finally, I want to tell you that I am so proud of you—something I believe many of us have not heard from our own parents. I am incredibly proud of you for opening yourself up to these pages and for being willing to do the hard work of facing yourself and your pain in order to find a way through. I hope that you can be proud of yourself for recognizing that your mental health is just as important as your physical health and that our generation is at a turning point at which we can change the narrative around the stigmas and taboos of mental health for future generations of Asian diasporas. You and I are part of a movement to destigmatize mental health, and our personal, intimate journeys are part of that greater collective shift. I hope this book is the beginning of your journey toward a life that is more empowered and authentic, and ultimately feels more like home.

Resources

Mental Health and Asian-Serving Organizations

AAPI Women Lead: imreadymovement.org

American Psychological Association: apa.org

Asian American Health Initiative: aahiinfo.org

Asian American Psychological Association: aapaonline.org

Asian American Suicide Prevention and Education: aaspe.net

Asian Mental Health Collective: asianmhc.org

Asian Mental Health Project: asianmentalhealthproject.com

Division 45: Society for the Psychological Study of Culture, Ethnicity, and Race: division45.org

Filipino Mental Health Initiative—San Mateo County: fmhi -smc.org

Mental Health America: mhanational.org

The Mental Health Coalition: thementalhealthcoalition.org

National Alliance on Mental Illness: nami.org

National Queer Asian Pacific Islander Alliance: nqapia.org

Red Canary Song: redcanarysong.net

South Asian Mental Health Initiative and Network: samhin.org

The Trevor Project: thetrevorproject.org

Therapist Directories

The Asian Australian Mental Health Practitioner List: just shapesandsounds.com/asianaustralianmhpractitionerlist

Asian Mental Health Collective (USA and Canada): asianmhc
   .org/apisaa, asianmhc.org/actd

Asians for Mental Health: asiansformentalhealth.com

The Black, African and Asian Therapy Network: baatn.org.uk

Inclusive Therapists: inclusivetherapists.com

South Asian Therapists: southasiantherapists.org

Asian-Focused Podcasts

Asianbossgirl: www.asianbossgirl.com

Asians Do Therapy: asiansdotherapy.com

Bamboo and Glass: bambooandglass.buzzsprout.com

Brownology: brownpsychologist.com/brownology

Dear Asian Americans: www.justlikemedia.com/show/dear-asian
   -americans

Books

Brackett, Marc. *Permission to Feel: Unlock the Power of Emotions to Help Yourself and Your Children Thrive* (Quercus, 2019).

Cacciatore, Joanne. *Bearing the Unbearable: Love, Loss, and the Heartbreaking Path of Grief* (Wisdom Publications, 2017).

Duckworth, Angela. *Grit: The Power of Passion and Perseverance* (Ebury Publishing, 2016).

Dweck, Carol. *Mindset: The New Psychology of Success* (Random House, 2006).

Eng, David L., and Shinhee Han. *Racial Melancholia, Racial Dissociation: On the Social and Psychic Lives of Asian Americans* (Duke University Press, 2019).

Hong, Cathy Park. *Minor Feelings: An Asian American Reckoning* (One World, 2020).

Lee, Erika. *The Making of Asian America: A History* (Simon and Schuster, 2015).

Menakem, Resmaa. *Grandmother's Hands: Racialized Trauma and the Pathway to Mending Our Hearts and Bodies* (Penguin, 2021).

Nagoski, Emily, and Amelia Nagoski. *Burnout: The Secret to Unlocking the Stress Cycle* (Ebury Publishing, 2019).

Stevenson, Howard C. *Promoting Racial Literacy in Schools: Differences That Make a Difference* (Teachers College Press, 2014).

Wijeyesinghe, Charmaine L., and Bailey W. Jackson III, eds. *New Perspectives on Racial Identity Development: A Theoretical and Practical Anthology* (NYU Press, 2001).

References

Bor, William, Angela J. Dean, Jacob Najman, and Reza Hayat-bakhsh. "Are Child and Adolescent Mental Health Problems Increasing in the 21st Century? A Systematic Review." *Australian and New Zealand Journal of Psychiatry* 48, no. 7 (2014): 606–616, https://doi.org/10.1177/0004867414533834.

Deci, E. L., R. Koestner, and R. M. Ryan. "A Meta-Analytic Review of Experiments Examining the Effects of Extrinsic Rewards on Intrinsic Motivation." Psychological Bulletin 125, no. 6 (1999): 627–668; discussion, 692–700, https://doi.org/10.1037/0033-2909.125.6.627.

Eng, David L., and Shinhee Han. *Racial Melancholia, Racial Dissociation: On the Social and Psychic Lives of Asian Americans.* Duke University Press, 2018.

Geiger, A.W., and Leslie Davis. "A Growing Number of American Teenagers—Particularly Girls—Are Facing Depression." Pew Research Center, July 12, 2019, https://www.pewresearch.org/fact-tank/2019/07/12/a-growing-number-of-american-teenagers-particularly-girls-are-facing-depression.

Isen, A. M., K. A. Daubman, and G. P. Nowicki. "Positive Affect Facilitates Creative Problem Solving." *Journal of Personal and Social Psychology* 52 (1987): 1122–1131, https://doi.org/10.1037/0022-3514.52.6.1122.

Kim, Claire Jean. "The Racial Triangulation of Asian Americans." *Politics and Society* 27, no. 1 (March 1999): 105–138, https://doi.org/10.1177/0032329299027001005.

Knopf, A. "Suicide Rates Increasing; Researchers Especially Worried about Teens." *Brown University Child and Adolescent Behavior Letter* 35 (2019): 9–10, https://doi.org/10.1002/cbl.30404.

Phelps, E. A. "Human Emotion and Memory: Interactions of the Amygdala and Hippocampal Complex." *Current Opinion in Neurobiology* 14 (2004): 198–202, https://doi.org/10.1016/j.conb.2004.03.015.

Shaver, T. K., J. E. Ozga, B. Zhu, et al. "Long-Term Deficits in Risky Decision-Making after Traumatic Brain Injury on a Rat Analog of the Iowa Gambling Task." *Brain Research* 1704 (2019): 103–113, https://doi.org/10.1016/j.brainres.2018.10.004.

Todd, R. M., M. R. Ehlers, D. J. Müller, et al. (2015). "Neurogenetic Variations in Norepinephrine Availability Enhance Perceptual Vividness." *Journal of Neuroscience* 35, no. 16 (2015): 6506–6516, https://doi.org/10.1523/JNEUROSCI.4489-14.2015.

Um, E., J. L. Plass, E. O. Hayward, and B. D. Homer. "Emotional Design in Multimedia Learning." *Journal of Educational Psychology* 104 (2012): 485–498, https://doi.org/10.1037/a0026609.

Vuilleumier, P. "How Brains Beware: Neural Mechanisms of Emotional Attention." *Trends in Cognitive Sciences* 9 (2005): 585–594, https://doi.org/10.1016/j.tics.2005.10.011.

Zadra, J. R., and G. L. Clore. "Emotion and Perception: The Role of Affective Information." *Wiley Interdisciplinary Reviews: Cognitive Science* 2, no. 6 (2011): 676–685, https://doi.org/10.1002/wcs.147.

Appendix

Examples of Core Values

Family
Ambition
Money
Health
Service
Community
Connection
Generosity
Authenticity
Fame
Adventure
Compassion
Honor
Courage
Dependability
Optimism
Loyalty
Perseverance
Integrity

Reliability
Independence
Education
Justice
Stewardship
Flexibility
Transparency
Empowerment
Creativity
Commitment
Passion
Impact
Respect
Beauty
Security
Balance
Personal Growth
Consistency
Fearlessness

Acknowledgments

This book came into existence because one person, my agent, Charles Kim, thought that I had something worthwhile to say and believed that Asian Americans needed more voices in the publishing world. Thank you for your unwavering confidence and encouragement throughout this entire journey. Heartfelt thank you to Nana K. Twumasi, my publisher and editor, whose compassionate and visionary guidance helped me write from a space of vulnerability that both terrified and freed me in the process. Thank you for your countless hours of editing and feedback that helped shape this book into what it is today.

Special thanks to my current and former colleagues, supervisors, teachers, and mentors, Richard Slatcher, Rebecca Bigler, Kathleen Saine, Deborah Wiebe, Skye Moffitt, Oscar Benitez, Kristi Baker, Virginia O'Hayer, Patrick Smith, Ashley Sanford, Andrea Pihlaskari, and Megan Brannan, all of whom left an indelible impact on my professional and personal identity and created safety for me in academic and professional spaces that seldom felt safe. I am grateful for each of you.

Thank you to my hype team, Lynn Kiang Wen, I-Fang Cheng, Angela Pan Wong, Sherry Oung, Nancy Lintakoon Kwan, Eve Choi, Michelle Son, Terri Le, Jennifer Choo, JoJo Luk, and Alice Morgan, who offered pep talks, encouragement, support, feedback, coffee, meals, and solace during the hardest months of my life and throughout the creation of this book. Thank you for your unfaltering belief that this book was possible and for holding me in compassion when I needed it most.

Thank you to my clients, who trusted me with their own journeys of self-discovery, empowerment, and freedom. Your courageous acts allowed me to believe that it was possible to wade into the pain and find that there was richness and hope on the other side. I am forever humbled and honored to walk with each of you and hope that I will be able to do this work until my last breath.

A big thank-you to my social media community, who supported me through the past two years of my life. From followers to fellow mental health advocates, professionals, activists, and content creators, thank you for growing with me and creating a community that has uplifted so many. Healing happens when we do it together.

To my extended family in Taiwan: Thank you for reminding me of who I am and the people I come from. Without your hospitality and our memories from my trips to Taiwan, I would not know what it meant to be filled with the strength and resilience of my ancestors.

A special thank-you to my parents, who bravely shared their own stories to help me understand what shaped them, which in turn shaped me. I am forever grateful for the seen and unseen ways in which you put my life ahead of your own and gifted me the privilege to choose a life that I could never have dreamed of. To my sister, Ellen Wang Tan, thank you for your steadfast encouragement and support throughout my entire life. I would be lost without you.

Thank you to my children, Evie and Theo, who patiently waited as I worked nights and weekends to finish this book and still received me with love and understanding when I was exhausted, irritable, and overwhelmed. Thank you for always teaching me about love, forgiveness, and the gifts of play and rest.

Finally, a million thanks to Jason Yeh, my life partner and co-conspirator. I am so lucky to get to build this life with you. Over this past year, you took the brunt of filling in all the gaps that this book caused in our family life. Thank you for always believing in me and encouraging me to reach for the stars. None of this would have been possible without you.

To the Spirit that moves above, within, and through us. Thank you for this gift of life and purpose.

Reading Group Guide

Discussion Questions

1. In chapter 1, Dr. Wang encourages us to be curious and question the frameworks that have thus far dictated how we show up in our lives. Acknowledging that outside our ingrained mindsets we may feel untethered or confused about how to make decisions, she introduces values-based living to help guide our questions and assist us to explore who we would like to be moving forward. Revisit your own core values. How do they point you toward a life that feels authentic and aligned with who you would like to be?

2. Some of us may experience guilt for acknowledging what we do not like about our lives or for being unhappy when our lives seem comparatively more privileged than those of our parents. Do you struggle to acknowledge your own unique hardships because they don't seem "as bad" as those your parents have encountered? How might you allow yourself to acknowledge that both your struggles and those

of your parents are valid and deserving of empathy and compassion?

3. In chapter 3, Dr. Wang explores some internalized messages we may have received about anger. What messages have you received about anger throughout your childhood and adult life? How have these messages shaped and changed how you approach your anger? How might your anger be trying to protect you?

4. Anger that goes unacknowledged and unnamed is pushed underground, where it can grow roots. Does this image resonate with you? Are there spaces in your life in which your unexpressed anger may have taken root and become rage? How do the effects of this appear in your life?

5. In chapter 4, we explore boundaries and how they allow us to stay connected with others while holding our own needs as an important part of the equation. How has your family of origin shaped how you relate to boundaries? How has your culture influenced how you relate to boundaries?

6. When you consider your relationship with your parents, has it ever felt more transactional versus relational? What are the currencies (attention, respect, achievement, wealth, or status, for example) that exist within this relationship? What do you wish this relationship might be like instead?

7. In chapter 8, Dr. Wang suggests that rest isn't something we earn; rather, rest serves as the fuel for future work, goals, and dreams. What models of rest and play did you have throughout your childhood? How have those models translated into your current life?

8. Dr. Wang introduces the idea of the "third space," a space "between worlds and within margins," often occupied by

children of immigrants and adoptees. Does this resonate with you? What might this third space represent to you?

9. Some of the losses that children of immigrants might experience can come through assimilation. What have you lost through assimilation? What has it cost you along the journey?

10. Can you share a goal you've been afraid to pursue because the fear of failure is so strong? Now consider how you might develop SMART goals (specific, measurable, achievable, realistic, and time-bound). Brainstorm with your community or reading group and consider the feedback that they offer as you build action steps to combat that fear.

About the Author

Dr. Jenny T. Wang is a Taiwanese American clinical psychologist and national speaker on the intersections of Asian American identity, mental health, and racial trauma. She received her doctorate from the University of Texas Southwestern Medical Center and completed her postdoctoral training at the Duke University Medical Center. Her professional mission is to destigmatize mental health within the Asian community and empower Asian Americans to prioritize their own mental well-being. In her private practice, she witnessed how difficult it was for Asian American clients to find mental health professionals who understand their unique immigrant and diasporic experiences. This led her to start mental health directories, including the Asians for Mental Health therapist directory (www.asiansformentalhealth.com), to connect individuals with culturally reverent mental health care for Asian American diasporas. She started the Instagram community Asians for Mental Health (@asiansformentalhealth), where she explores the unique ways in which Asian American identity impacts our mental health. She lives in Houston, Texas, with her family.